SUPERSTITION

SUPERSTITION

Belief in the Age of Science

Robert L. Park

Princeton University Press
Princeton and Oxford

REQUESTS FOR PERMISSION TO REPRODUCE MATERIAL
FROM THIS WORK SHOULD BE SENT TO
PERMISSIONS, PRINCETON UNIVERSITY PRESS

PUBLISHED BY PRINCETON UNIVERSITY PRESS,
41 WILLIAM STREET, PRINCETON, NEW JERSEY 08540

IN THE UNITED KINGDOM: PRINCETON UNIVERSITY PRESS,
6 OXFORD STREET, WOODSTOCK, OXFORDSHIRE OX20 1TW

PRESS.PRINCETON.EDU

SECOND PRINTING, AND FIRST PAPERBACK PRINTING, 2010
PAPERBACK ISBN: 978-0-691-14597-6

THE LIBRARY OF CONGRESS HAS CATALOGED THE CLOTH EDITION OF
THIS BOOK AS FOLLOWS

PARK, ROBERT L.
SUPERSTITION : BELIEF IN THE AGE OF SCIENCE / ROBERT L. PARK.—1ST ED.
P.   CM.
INCLUDES BIBLIOGRAPHICAL REFERENCES.
ISBN 978-0-691-13355-3 (CLOTH : ALK. PAPER)
1. RELIGION AND SCIENCE.   2. RELIGION AND SOCIOLOGY.
3. BELIEF AND DOUBT.   I. TITLE.
BL240.3.P37 2008
215—DC22   2008014926

BRITISH LIBRARY CATALOGING-IN-PUBLICATION DATA IS AVAILABLE

THIS BOOK HAS BEEN COMPOSED IN UNIVERS AND SABON

PRINTED ON ACID-FREE PAPER. ∞

PRINTED IN THE UNITED STATES OF AMERICA

3   5   7   9   10   8   6   4   2

CONTENTS

Introduction: Lessons from a tree   vii

CHAPTER ONE
A BIGGER PRIZE   1
In which we discover scientists of faith

CHAPTER TWO
THE SECRET OF LIFE   23
*In which Darwin's theory of evolution by natural
selection survives*

CHAPTER THREE
MIRACLE AT COLUMBIA   56
In which both sides pray for victory

CHAPTER FOUR
GIVING UP THE GHOST   79
In which we search for the soul

CHAPTER FIVE
THE SILENT ARMY   93
In which we search for an afterlife

CHAPTER SIX
THE TSUNAMI GOD   104
In which the innocent suffer

CHAPTER SEVEN
THE NEW AGE   116
In which anything goes

CONTENTS

CHAPTER EIGHT
SCHRÖDINGER'S GRAVE   129
In which quantum mysticism is found to be superstition

CHAPTER NINE
THE BARBARY DUCK   142
In which the body heals itself

CHAPTER TEN
THE DEER   161
In which the placebo effect is explained

CHAPTER ELEVEN
THE MORAL LAW   188
In which we instinctively know right from wrong

CHAPTER TWELVE
THE LAST BUTTERFLY   202
In which there is no place else to go

Bibliography   217

Index   221

INTRODUCTION

Lessons from a tree

Almost a year had passed since the tree had fallen, but it was not hard to find. A large red oak almost three feet in diameter, its roots had pulled out of the soft ground on the steep slope of the ravine after a week of heavy rain. It hit the ground with such impact that the heavy trunk snapped in two. The broken end of the trunk still pointed straight down the slope, reaching almost to the edge of the trail. The rest had been cut up and carted off to clear the trail. I had imagined that seeing the tree might evoke some memory of that day, but there was nothing. It was just a fallen tree, like all the other fallen trees that slowly rot on the forest floor.

The doctors had given me the green light to try jogging, but it seemed much harder here than on a treadmill in the National Rehabilitation Center. I was still panting when two elderly men walked briskly down the trail. Seeing me looking at the fallen tree, they paused. "You know," one of them said, "when that tree fell, it fell on a guy."

"Yeah," I said, "I know. I was the guy." They looked stunned.

"We never knew what had happened to you," the other said, his voice breaking and his eyes filling with tears, "I have prayed for you every night since."

It was my first contact with anyone who had been a witness to what took place that day. David O'Connor and Shaun McCarty are Catholic priests. Former faculty in a nearby seminary, they would meet almost every day to walk this peaceful trail beside Northwest Branch, once a millstream, both for the exercise and to share each other's company. Two years earlier, on a Sunday afternoon, they were on their walk when the tree fell.

They were not the first to find me; an undocumented Salvadoran immigrant had already called 911 on his cell phone. Not knowing the extent of my injuries, the three of them were afraid to try to free me. Other people came by and paused, but reluctant to get involved, hurried on. The man with the cell phone called 911 again to ask what was keeping them. The ambulance, it seems, could go only as far as the historic Old Adelphi Mill. The fallen tree was still a half mile further down the trail. Seeing no sign of anyone at the mill, the rescue team thought it must have been a crank call and returned to the fire station. When the second call came in, they hurried back, searching farther down the trail on foot. I have a single fragmentary memory of someone writing in a notebook, walking beside the litter as they carried me back to the mill and the waiting ambulance. I gave him my name and home phone number, and lapsed back into unconsciousness.

Before the rescue team arrived, David O'Conner and Shaun McCarty did what priests know how to do—they administered the last rites of the Church. Only a few years earlier, prayer would have been all anyone could have done. Even the cell phone the Salvadoran immigrant used to call 911 was a very new technology at the time. A massive infection from soil bacteria that had entered my body cavity by way of numerous compound fractures was the major threat. It responded only to massive doses of a newly developed antibiotic infused daily into the vena cava of my heart by means of a catheter inserted through a vein in the arm. The Washington National Hospital Center used a modern medical-imaging device to thread the catheter all the way to my heart. I would not be telling the story had it not been for recent advances in medicine and technology.

Standing there beside the fallen oak, we shared what we knew of that day. The two priests invited me to join them on the rest of their walk. In the months and years that followed I would meet with David and Shaun a few times each week to walk with them beside that woodland stream.

I am a scientist and a professor of physics at a major public university. I am also a husband, a grandfather, a veteran of the Korean War, and an atheist. Now in my late seventies and grateful to be still alive, I found myself developing a friendship with two retired Irish-American Catholic priests. Aside from compassion for the human condition, we seemed to have little in common. We had followed very different roads, and ended up with very different beliefs. Those beliefs gave us much to talk about.

My conversations with these wise and gentle men of faith began the intellectual process that eventually led to this book. Walk with us now along that wooded path beside the millstream and we'll talk about belief.

CHAPTER ONE

A BIGGER PRIZE

In which we discover scientists of faith

Emerging from the limousine, Charles Townes might have paused for just a moment if his eyes, still sharp at eighty-nine, had caught the characteristic flutter of a butterfly's wings. Years of butterfly collecting trains the eye and the brain to pick out that distinctive movement among the clutter of images carried by the optic nerve—and Townes had collected butterflies since he was a schoolboy in South Carolina. It was early spring in London and it would not be surprising if a Camberwell beauty (*Nymphalis antiopa*) had sought a perch on the west face of Buckingham Palace, where it could bask in the afternoon sun. Butterflies generate too little internal heat to fly. They spend time basking in the sun with their wings spread to collect the heat needed for flight.

Usually the first large butterfly seen in the spring, *Nymphalis antiopa* stirs the heart of every lepidopterist. It's a signal to get out the net and keep it close at hand in case a good specimen is spotted. Called a mourning cloak in North America because of its resemblance to the traditional cloak worn at funerals, the dark wings of *Nymphalis antiopa* are bordered with ivory. Field guides list it among "black" butterflies, but up close in sunlight the dark wings are a deep reddish-brown with a row of tiny blue dots beside the ivory borders.

As a boy, Charles had imagined becoming an entomologist and collecting every butterfly on earth. His father was a lawyer, but the family lived on a small farm on the edge of Greenville, South Carolina, and when his chores were done, Charles often wandered the woods and fields with a butterfly net on his shoulder. However, as he approached college age, Charles recalls, he decided that "my older brother Henry was so much better at it than I that I thought I had to do something else." Henry did go on to become a noted entomologist, while Charles turned to physics, inventing the maser, which in turn led to the laser. Although he still collects butterflies for pleasure, Professor Townes, already one of the most honored scientists in the world, was not at Buckingham Palace to collect butterflies, but for the formal awarding of the Templeton Prize by the Duke of Edinburgh. The Templeton Prize for Progress Toward Research or Discoveries about Spiritual Realities is the largest annual financial award given to an individual for intellectual accomplishment.

SPIRITUAL REALITIES

The monetary value of the prize, now about $1.5 million dollars, is adjusted annually to ensure that it is always larger than the Nobel Prize. According to the John Templeton Foundation, that reflects Sir John Templeton's conviction that research directed toward spiritual realities could bring even greater benefits to humankind than technology-directed research. It also reflects his conviction that money makes things happen.

It certainly works for Templeton. Frequently described as a humble man in spite of his staggering wealth, he can afford to be humble. He became a billionaire by pioneering the use of globally diversified mutual funds. He was born into a middle-class family in the Bible-Belt town of Winchester, Kentucky; his parents, devout Presbyterians, emphasized the virtues of thrift and compassion. He learned both lessons so well that in 1968 he renounced his U.S. citizenship and moved to the Bahamas, becoming a British citizen to avoid the U.S. income tax. He was knighted by the Queen in 1987 for his philanthropies. Sir John Templeton still resides in the Bahamas, and of course he still pays no U.S. taxes.

MINORITY REPORT

Perhaps the most honored scientist of our time, Townes shared the 1964 Nobel Prize for fundamental discoveries in quantum electronics, culminating in the development of the maser and the laser—inventions that have had an enormous impact on science and society. He was awarded the National Medal of Science by President Ronald Reagan in 1982 and has gathered numerous other awards and prizes.

Born and raised in a devoutly Baptist household in a Bible-Belt town not unlike Templeton's home town, Townes, like Templeton, remained devout his entire life and still begins and ends every day with a prayer.

A graduate of Furman, a local Baptist college, Townes was from the beginning drawn to science. But the amount and quality of the science offered at Furman was limited, so he took a degree in modern languages and went on to Duke for an MA in physics. At Duke his extraordinary ability in physics was recognized, and he was encouraged to go on to Caltech for his PhD. At Caltech he endured a certain amount of teasing for his religious beliefs, not only from fellow students but from William Smythe, his thesis advisor. In an interview with Tim Radford of *The Guardian* sixty-five years later, he recalled being chided by Smythe, "Charlie you can't know that Jesus was the son of God." Townes resented it—and he still does.

A few years later, by now a faculty member at Columbia, Townes joined the Men's Group at the famed Riverside Church in New York. Since few scientists ever attend church, he was asked to talk to the group about his views. He titled his talk "The Convergence of Science and Religion." The editor of

Think magazine, published by IBM, heard the talk and liked it so much he published it in the April 1966 issue. The editor of the *MIT Alumni Journal* a nonscientist like the editor of *Think*, liked it so much he reprinted it. But while magazine editors may have liked it, many of their scientist readers did not, and it drew complaints from scientists and prominent MIT alumni. Half a century later, in a statement at the Templeton Prize news conference, Townes recalled these slights: "It reflected a common view among many scientists at the time that one could not be a scientist and also be religiously oriented. There was an antipathy towards discussion of spirituality."

The antipathy has not softened. Indeed, with the rise of religion-inspired terrorism and antiscience religious fundamentalism around the world, antipathy toward religion among scientists has hardened into direct confrontation. By 2006 there was at least one antireligion title by a prominent scientist in the *New York Times* nonfiction best-seller list every week.

"The Convergence of Science and Religion" was cited by the judges in awarding the Templeton Prize. Their report quoted a single line: "Understanding the order in the universe and understanding the purpose of the universe are not identical, but they are also not very far apart."

They are a universe apart. Science and religion are on divergent paths, growing ever farther apart as knowledge expands. Most religious scientists consciously partition their lives, relying on scientific reasoning on one side of the partition and revelation on the other. Townes appears to partition his life the same way, but without quite being aware that he's doing it. On the science side he applies logic and reason to great effect. But on the religion side, since Scripture provides the answers, he ends up redefining words to make the two views of the universe appear to be coming together.

His phrase, "the purpose of the universe," moreover is rather scary. "Purpose" conjures up images of fanaticism. Once people convince themselves that they have been put on Earth as instruments in some divine plan, there seems to be no limit to the horrors they are willing to commit to carry out that plan. In his beautiful *Dreams of a Final Theory*, Steven Weinberg, another great Nobel-laureate physicist and an avowed atheist, expressed quite a different view: "The more the universe seems comprehensible, the more it seems pointless."

Many nonscientists have criticized Weinberg for this line; scientists, however, generally find a purposeless existence to be wonderfully liberating—we are free to establish our own goals and to venture across any intellectual boundaries without looking for no-trespassing signs. Humans are free to decide what kind of world we want to live in, and science has given us the tools to set about the business of building that world. *Naturalism* is the idea that scientific laws are the only way to explain the world. As we enter the third millennium, naturalism is the dominant philosophy of scientists. But it is not the philosophy of Charles Townes.

THE FAITHFUL SCIENTIST

"Many people don't realize that science basically involves faith," Townes said in his Templeton Prize news conference. Townes had made that point many times before. On questions of laser physics I would happily defer to Townes, but this is a matter of the English language. Here we must defer to the dictionaries. He is confusing two very different meanings of the word "faith." Pick your dictionary; they all list at least two quite different meanings. In the *Concise Oxford English Dictionary* that I keep on my desk:

> faith n.   1 complete trust or confidence.   2 strong belief in a religion, based on spiritual conviction rather than proof.

Some dictionaries break it down into finer variations, but these two meanings are all I need to make my point: scientists use the word "faith" to express their confidence that the laws of nature will prevail, beginning with the law of cause and effect. The religious use of "faith" implies belief in a higher power that makes things happen independent of a physical cause. This defines superstition. The two meanings of "faith" are thus not only different, they are exact opposites.

Science is conditional: when better experimental evidence becomes available, scientists revise their picture of the universe to fit the facts. Our senses may at times deceive us, as when we see a mirage in the desert. A scientist would say the way to avoid being deceived by a mirage is to understand the laws of optics, enabling us to invent instruments that let us see more clearly, perhaps a polarized lens. Much of the work of science consists of refining the methods of observation to avoid being deceived, including self-deception. Nature is the only arbiter. Religion, by contrast, may call on the faithful to deny the evidence of their senses if it disagrees with Holy Scripture. It's hard to imagine that anyone as careful as Townes could have confused the two meanings of faith over and over again without consulting a dictionary.

Nevertheless, the scientist in Townes is clearly dominant. He places Darwin's theory of natural selection above Genesis as an explanation for the origin of humans. While he may think of himself as a Baptist, pray twice a day, and attend church every Sunday, as a scientist he recognizes that the authors of the Bible could not have understood the scientific implications of their words. To make the Bible agree with his scientific conclusions, Townes interprets the Bible metaphorically, as do virtually all religious scientists. Southern Baptists who are nonscientists, however, are inclined to interpret the Bible quite literally.

Townes was not the first physicist to receive the Templeton Prize. Before 2001, however, the name of the prize was simply the "Templeton Prize for Progress in Religion," and the winners were mostly celebrities drawn from the religious world, beginning with Mother Teresa in 1973. Predictably, the evangelist Billy Graham was a winner, receiving the prize in 1982. Even Charles Colson, whose celebrity status came as a result of his conviction in the Watergate scandal, was awarded the prize in 1993 as the founder of a prison ministry called the Prison Fellowship. The first real physicist to win the prize was Paul Davies in 1995. An Australian, Davies is best known for his science popularizations, including *The Mind of God: The Scientific Basis for a Rational World* in 1992.

Templeton's thinking about the prize seems to have been evolving. It went to another physicist, Ian Barbour, in 1999, and two years later the name of the prize was changed to the Templeton Prize for Progress Toward Research or Discoveries about Spiritual Realities. Most of the recipients since have been, as Richard Dawkins scathingly put it in *The God Delusion*, scientists who "say something nice about religion." Most of them have been physicists or cosmologists.

BUYING A DIALOG

Ian Barbour's PhD was from the University of Chicago, where he was a teaching assistant to Enrico Fermi, the great Italian physicist who fled fascist Italy with his Jewish wife at the start of World War II. Fermi carried out the first atomic chain reaction beneath the university of Chicago stadium, ensuring that the United States and not Nazi Germany would build the atomic bomb first. Barbour completed his PhD in 1949, and seemed headed for a career as one of the leaders of American physics along with other scientists from the Manhattan Project. But two years later he enrolled in Yale Divinity School, earning a divinity degree in 1956. He became a professor in both physics and religion at Carleton College in Minnesota, and was highly regarded in both fields. Like virtually all religious scientists, Barbour flatly rejects the literal interpretation of the biblical story of Genesis by the creationists, seeing it as clearly metaphorical. He is credited with having created the contemporary dialogue between science and religion.

The importance of Barbour's dialog was recognized by Sir John Templeton from the beginning. While Templeton may genuinely believe the Christian myth, he also respects science.

Why shouldn't he? The scientific revolution, after all, led to the fantastic growth in the world economy that made him a billionaire. Perhaps Templeton believes God has chosen him to show the world that, as he put it, theology and science are two windows onto the same landscape. It would follow that if scientists could be persuaded to delve into religion, it would benefit both religion and science. How then should he go about convincing scientists of this?

Why not just buy the dialogue between science and religion? Templeton proceeded to do exactly that. After all, there's no point in being super rich if you can't throw your weight around. It was easier to buy the dialog than you might imagine. The machinery was already in place. The John Templeton Foundation had been created in 1987 to serve as catalyst for scientific studies into the "Big Questions." These are questions about such things as the nature of consciousness and the origin of life that seemed unanswerable in 1987. They form the basis of Barbour's dialogue. The Foundation now gives away about $60 million in research grants each year. Recipients often feel moved to express their gratitude by inventing some sort of common ground between science and religion, thus reinforcing the myth of convergence. The Foundation even bought a magazine, *Science & Spirit,* and devoted it to publicizing the dialogue.

The biggest coup was to go directly to the staff of the American Association for the Advancement of Science with an offer of a million dollars to create The AAAS Dialogue between Science and Religion. The AAAS couldn't resist. One million dollars still sounds like a lot of money to scientists. Indeed, anywhere there is the sound of a dialogue between science and religion, it's a safe bet that Templeton's people are there handing out money. What he has bought with his money are elaborate sound effects meant to create an illusion that science and religion are finding common ground. However, it's an illusion that has been shattered by the muffled sound of explosions as religious fanatics blow up themselves and total strangers with the goal of replacing civilization with Islamic rule.

Perhaps the most ambitious dialogue was a three-day discussion in May, 1999, of "Cosmic Questions," held at the Smithsonian Institute in Washington DC. It was cosponsored by the AAAS, but the money came from Templeton. Ian Barbour, however, was not there. He was on his way to Buckingham Palace to receive the 1999 Templeton Prize.

The featured event was an exchange between Sir John Polkinghorne and Steven Weinberg, presenting contrasting views on the question: Is the universe designed? Both are physicists who have contributed to particle theory, but the similarity ends there. Weinberg, who shared the 1979 Nobel Prize for the unification of electromagnetism and the weak force, is an avowed atheist. Polkinghorne, like Weinberg, was a theoretical particle physicist. He made significant contributions to the discovery of the quark. However, in 1981 he resigned his physics professorship at Cambridge to study for the ministry in the Church of England, and became an ordained Anglican priest in 1982.

Is the universe designed? "No" was the eloquent title of Weinberg's talk. It came within one letter of being the shortest of all possible titles. The laws of nature, Weinberg said, are "cold and impersonal." Noting that his invitation described the conference as "a constructive dialogue between science and religion," Weinberg growled that "I favor a dialogue, but not a constructive one." Although physicists generally agreed that Weinberg came out the clear winner, they didn't have a vote. But Sir John Templeton did—the 2002 Templeton Prize was awarded to Rev. John Polkinghorne.

THE ANTHROPIC PRINCIPLE

Polkinghorne countered Weinberg's naturalism by describing the universe as "shot through with signs of mind." Had the fundamental constants that show up in the laws of physics been even slightly different, he argued, the universe as we know it would not exist. This is the so-called "anthropic principle," which is often defined as meaning that the universe has been fine-tuned to make life possible. But just how finely tuned is it? It's like saying the universe is big. Compared to what?

Six of the next seven recipients of the Templeton Prize would be physicists or cosmologists, beginning with Ian Barbour who, as we said, was on his way to Buckingham Palace to accept the 1999 Templeton Prize while Polkinghorne and Weinberg carried on the dialog. All eight Templeton Prize-winning physicists cite the anthropic principle as evidence, if not proof, that the universe was designed for life. The designer would presumably qualify as God.

Eventually, the Templeton Prize would be awarded to John Barrow, a British cosmologist who, with Frank Tipler, literally wrote the book in 1986 on the anthropic principle, *The Anthropic Cosmological Principle*. But what does the anthropic principle actually say? In his debate with Steven Weinberg, Sir John Polkinghorne used the most popular version, sometimes referred to as the strong anthropic principle:

> The fundamental parameters of the universe are such as to permit the creation of observers within it.

I would be inclined to state it a little less pretentiously. Borrowing from the style of Yogi Berra, it might be written:

> If things were different, things would not be the way things are.

If that doesn't strike you as terribly deep, you may not be suitable material for a Templeton Prize. Nevertheless, the anthropic principle is so widely invoked as evidence for intelligent design that we should take a few minutes to examine its logic little more closely.

THE INHOSPITABLE UNIVERSE

In their 2001 analysis of the anthropic principle, "Probabilities and the Fine-Tuning Argument: A Skeptical View," Timothy

McGrew, Lydia McGrew, and Eric Vestrup, writing in *Mind*, invoke "The Principle of Indifference: it is unreasonable to suggest that any one range of values for the constants is more probable a priori than any other similar range."

If the universe was designed for life, it must be said that it is a shockingly inefficient design. There are vast reaches of the universe in which life as we know it is clearly impossible: gravitational forces would be crushing, or radiation levels are too high for complex molecules to exist, or temperatures would make the formation of stable chemical bonds impossible. Even in our own solar system it seems increasingly likely that Earth is the only outpost of life. The search for life to which we are not related—extraterrestrial life—is perhaps the greatest quest of science, but so far it has been disappointing. Fine-tuned for life? It would make more sense to ask why God designed a universe so inhospitable to life.

At this point I can hear the voices of David O'Conner and Shaun McCarty sternly admonishing me in the course of one of our contemplative walks beside Northwest Branch that "God's ways are not our ways. We cannot know his reasons." (David and Shaun, I remind you, are the two Catholic priests who prayed for me as I lay pinned beneath that tree.)

David and Shaun were right. "God" is sometimes used by physicists as a collective term for the imperfectly understood forces of nature. But the fine-tuning argument is an example of the "Texas-sharpshooter fallacy": The sharpshooter fires his six-gun at the side of a barn, and then walks over and draws a bull's-eye around the bullet hole. We will encounter other examples of this fallacy in later chapters. Was it fine-tuning that caused that tree to fall as I ran by? This is not a very useful way to think about the world.

The only thing the anthropic principle makes clear is that we do not yet have a theory explaining why the fundamental constants are what they are. There are, of course, many things we can't explain, but the list grows shorter daily. It might be well to remind ourselves that for 99.8% of the time that our species has existed, nobody on Earth knew or cared that such things as fundamental constants even existed. The fundamental constants are now at the very heart of modern physics.

There are still great problems out there for physicists to solve. Sometime in the coming years I expect it will be found that the fundamental constants are not so fundamental—that they emerge naturally from more fundamental laws. They have the values they do, we will find, because they cannot have any other values. That's exciting if you're a young physicist looking to make a mark. It's less comforting if you're an aging physicist running out of time to find out how the story ends. Invoking a designer solves nothing. It only raises the additional question of where the designer came from.

DISSENT

Not everyone was happy about the American Association for the Advancement of Science (AAAS) selling its soul to Templeton. Why had the most important scientific organization in America, perhaps in the world, allowed the voice of antiscience to assume the guise of a dialog between science and religion?

AAAS occupies a unique position among scientific societies in that it fosters the entire spectrum of scientific research. The weekly journal of the AAAS, *Science,* covers an eclectic mix of technical scientific papers in virtually every discipline, along with news and opinion covering the interaction of science and society. Because *Science* is such a popular source of science news, and because subscribers are automatically made members of the AAAS, membership is huge and includes many interested laymen as well as many lapsed scientists. In addition to individual members, AAAS also has many powerful organizational members, such as the American Chemical Society, the American Physical Society, and the American Society of Cell Biologists.

In addition to special meetings such as the Cosmic Questions Conference, AAAS holds a huge annual meeting, which is brilliantly arranged to coincide with the annual meeting of the Association of Science Writers, guaranteeing heavy media coverage. Because of its large membership, and the fact that *Science* is a major source of news stories for the media, AAAS wields substantial political clout.

The AAAS is precious to the scientific community. The fact that a single individual had been able to buy a major AAAS program for his own purposes was disturbing to many members. For whatever cultural reason, it was the physicists on the AAAS Council, of whom I was one, who seemed to feel most strongly that religion was playing far too great a role in the affairs of the AAAS. The outgoing president of the AAAS at that time was the late Stephen Jay Gould, a highly respected, even beloved, paleontologist whose position on the science/religion nexus would be best described as "separate but equal."

DIFFERENT LANDSCAPES

Gould recognized the spiritual nature of *Homo sapiens* and argued that although religion and science are both necessary to a full life, by their nature they cannot be reconciled. He revived the archaic term "magesteria" to describe these nonoverlapping domains of human existence. The magesteria of science and that of religion view the world through different windows, but unlike Templeton's analogy of windows that give you different views of the same landscape, Gould's windows look out on totally different landscapes. Experiment is the window of science; the window of religion is revelation. They see very different universes. Both, Gould argued, are worthy of respect but our institutions must be structured to keep them separate; which, of course, is also what the First Amendment to the Constitution seeks to do. The principle of nonoverlapping magesteria is contrary to Townes's belief that science and religion are converging, and a denial of Templeton's dream that science will confirm his Christian religious beliefs. The AAAS Dialogue between Science and Religion seemed destined to be unproductive and divisive—and so it has been.

Unfortunately, Stephen Jay Gould, who had the stature and personal charm to deal with both sides, also had to deal with cancer. He died in the spring of 2002. In the never-ending struggle against those who turn to religious myths instead of science to explain why things are the way they are, science had lost one of its most eloquent and beloved champions. Pain from the cancer that finally claimed his life never dimmed his sense of humor nor lessened his fierce determination to tell the story of evolution with such clarity and logic that people could not help but understand.

For many years Gould had carried on a sometimes-sharp exchange with Richard Dawkins, the other great expositor of evolution in our time, over the role of what Gould called "punctuated equilibrium," or the observation that evolution sometimes occurs in spurts separated by periods of relative stasis. The dispute was fairly technical and was only over the degree to which evolution occurs through punctuated equilibrium as opposed to gradualism. Although both Gould and Dawkins championed evolution, evolution deniers sought to use the dispute to argue that the evolutionists couldn't even agree among themselves.

Actually, the open dispute between these renowned champions of evolution was a classic example of how science arrives at ever-closer descriptions of the truth. Science is a wide-open shoot-out in which the weapons are scientific data. The side with the best evidence wins. Nothing is sacred—faith is scorned. Dawkins disparaged Gould's proposal to regard science and religion as nonoverlapping magesteria (often abbreviated as NOMA). In Dawkins view, any agreement that science and religion refrain from commenting on each others' realm would simply provide cover for indefensible religious claims.

Unfortunately, the AAAS never dealt satisfactorily with the issues raised by the Dialog between Science and Religion. A compromise was reached under which the John Templeton

Foundation would supply less than half of the program's budget. That may have constrained the power of Templeton to dictate the agenda, but it did nothing to address the question of principle: should the American Association for the Advancement of Science solicit or accept large gifts designated for purposes other than the advancement of science? Many scientists believe strongly that it should not.

SHEDDING YOUR SKIN

The winners of the Templeton Prize and Templeton himself all seem to have been raised in strongly religious households. I generally find the same pattern among those of my physics colleagues who remain religious. Their religious convictions were being instilled in them even as they learned to speak. They are no more likely to shed their religion after puberty than they are to stop thinking in their first tongue. It happens, but not often. H. L. Mencken once grumbled that he could never trust an atheist who was raised as a Catholic—eventually they revert to their childhood faith. I doubt if Mencken had any hard data to back up his assertion, but everyone can recall anecdotes that illustrate the power of early childhood indoctrination. We can't help it—we are prisoners of our upbringing. But that's only part of the story: we are also prisoners of our genetic inheritance. The combination produces a few surprises.

Francis Collins, a geneticist at NIH and the director of the National Human Genome Research Institute, is such a surprise. Chosen in 2002 to replace James Watson, the discoverer of the structure of DNA, as head of the project, Collins does not fit the usual pattern. He grew up on a small farm in the Shenandoah Valley of Virginia that lacked indoor plumbing, but his parents were not farmers; they simply did not place a high value on material possessions. His father held a PhD in English and was a drama professor at Mary Baldwin College. His mother was a playwright. Together they produced summer plays on a stage built on the farm, resulting in a stream of interesting and lively summer visitors. The summers were a joy for Francis, but it was not easy in the winter. There were stock to be taken care of and outdoor chores. Inside there were lessons.

Because she was not satisfied with the quality of the public schools, his mother schooled Francis at home through the sixth grade. Home schooling seemed to serve Francis well. He entered college at the University of Virginia at sixteen and went on to a PhD in physical chemistry at Yale, and entered medical school at the University of North Carolina.

Collins describes his parents as "nominally Christian," but religion was certainly not an important part of their life. Indeed, Francis regarded himself as an atheist through college. After all, in a field like physical chemistry that's the norm. Like his parents, religion had not seemed very important, and he never thought seriously about the evidence for or against belief. At age twenty-seven, in his third year of medical school and encountering patients who relied heavily on their faith to cope with their suffering, Francis Collins finally began to think about religion.

In the first chapter of his 2006 book, *The Language of God*, Collins relates a visit to a neighbor who was a Methodist minister to ask "whether faith made any logical sense." By then in his late twenties, Francis Collins was clearly searching for something. Was he expecting to engage a Methodist minister in a debate? Having asked similar questions of Methodist ministers at a much earlier age, I would have warned him that it wasn't going to happen. However, the minister handled it well, hearing him out and then giving him a copy of the C. S. Lewis book *Mere Christianity* to read. Perhaps all Christian ministers today are taught in seminary to refer the wavering to C. S. Lewis.

I must tell you straight out that I am no fan of C. S. Lewis, although I do admire the way he employs the English language to tell entertaining children's stories. We even gave a copy of

Narnia to our grandsons. After all, they enjoyed Harry Potter without being corrupted into believing in magic. They like stories, but they learned early that they're only stories.

A close friend we have known since college remained single and devoted her entire life to teaching elementary school. She was very smart, very caring, and totally dedicated to opening the children's eyes to the world. They were incredibly lucky to have her for a teacher, but a lifetime of talking to first graders left her handicapped in talking to adults. Lewis has the same problem. His logic is better suited to children than adults. He likes to put his arguments in the form of multiple-choice questions with no right answers. Because an animal is neither a sheep nor a goat, does not mean it's a cow. And even if every straw man set up by Lewis is an idiot, that's not evidence that Jesus was God.

The important idea that Collins took away from *Mere Christianity* was the concept of the "moral law." C. S. Lewis was certainly not the first to observe that people instinctively know right from wrong, nor, as we will see, was he the last.

BEING HUMAN

Toward the end of his book Collins relates a very moving experience in the summer of 1989. Just a year shy of forty, he had traveled to Nigeria as a volunteer to a small mission hospital, freeing the hospital staff to attend their annual conference. While treating a young African farmer suffering from advanced tuberculosis, Collins had an overwhelming religious experience. He interpreted it as a vision of God's purpose. A PhD chemist with a medical degree besides, Francis Collins must surely be aware of the extent to which our emotions are influenced by hormones secreted in response to instructions from the brain. That this brilliant scientist would not recognize his own religious experience as a hormone rush is evidence of the controlling power of our brain chemistry. While we may recognize the role of hormones in others, it is much harder to make the connection when it happens to us. It seems that hormones have the power not only to turn on your emotions, but to turn off your critical faculties at the same time. Little wonder that we humans are virtually helpless in the face of a concerted hormone assault.

My students are uneasy when the chemical manipulation of emotions comes up in class. They are having their own hormonal problems. I try to reassure them that this is perfectly normal. We share many of our hormonal responses with pre-human and even pre-mammalian ancestors. It's perfectly normal and even essential to our survival. It's important for them to recognize, however, that these responses evolved to aid survival in a Pleistocene wilderness. As members of a civilized society we have an obligation to try to understand our impulses and not follow them blindly.

As an example, I share with them that I have been married to the same woman for fifty-seven years. I have no doubt that at our first meeting in a college library our pheromones matched receptors in each other's olfactory system. Pheromones are nature's panderers, but they are not completely promiscuous. To keep you from getting excited by your own pheromones, they do not attach to your own receptors. Nor do they attach to the receptors of closely related people such as siblings, who produce similar pheromones. This adaptation has the effect of discouraging inbreeding.

You are not conscious of "smelling" pheromones because the signal from your pheromone receptors is routed straight to the amygdalae, bypassing the cerebral cortex. The amygdalae respond by calling on the hypothalamus to release arousal hormones, testosterone and estrogen, as well as adrenalin, into the bloodstream. If the person smiles at you, the hormone mix you generate may include norepinephrine, which is so hard to pronounce that it's often called noradrenalin. Noradrenalin synthesizes the formation of synapses in the brain, thereby enabling you to remember everything that's going on, including a lot of irrelevant detail. From that time on, merely thinking about the other person or hearing the other person's voice on the telephone produces an effect similar to the pheromones. The amygdalae are reminded of the original encounter and instruct the hypothalamus to release a cocktail of hormones that mimics the mix of hormones during that memorable meeting. Noradrenalin is responsible for the vivid memories you retain of everything that was going on around you when you heard the news about 9/11 or that the Chicago Cubs had won the Series, if that's what's important to you.

As the relationship develops, the hormone mix may begin to include oxytocin, a tiny peptide molecule that plays a large role in human emotions related to reproduction, particularly emotions other than simple lust, such as mothering. Each time there is a satisfying interaction with the person, the level of oxytocin tends to rise. Oxytocin induces the deeper feelings of love and loyalty associated with lasting relationships.

By this point my students are squirming. I have just reduced the most meaningful parts of their lives to chemistry. "No matter," I reassure them, "you will discover that understanding what is actually going on won't make it any less wonderful; if anything it will enrich the experience. You will marvel, as every scientist should, at what natural selection can accomplish. Just enjoy it." It's the complex interaction of many factors working together—sensory input, synaptic connections in the brain, memory storage, the endocrine system, and conditioned responses. Together they make the experience uniquely personal. Does all this raise questions of free will? Of course it does.

SACRED DISHONESTY

Although Francis Collins cannot be unaware of the power of a hormone rush to induce a religious experience, he has chosen to compartmentalize his world, as religious scientists must. Scientific interpretation of religious experience is left outside the door, lest it intrude on spiritual explanations. Interviewed by *New York Times* writer Cornelia Dean, Walt Ruloff, producer of the creationist-inspired movie *Expelled* commented that genome researchers who find evidence suggestive of design in their research may be afraid to report it because it conflicts with the mainline view. He cited Dr. Collins as an example. It's difficult to imagine Francis Collins being afraid of anything, so Dean called Collins and asked him directly about Ruloff's statement. He was not afraid to tell her that Ruloff's remarks were "ridiculous."

They were more than ridiculous. Ruloff appears to have been engaging in the all-too-common practice of "sacred dishonesty". But lies in the name of God are still lies. "From a biologist's perspective," Collins wrote in *The Language of God*, "the evidence in favor of evolution is utterly compelling. Darwin's theory of natural selection provides a fundamental framework for understanding the relationships of all living things. The predictions of evolution have been borne out in more ways than Darwin could have possibly imagined when he proposed his theory 150 years ago, especially in the field of genomics."

Speaking to a national gathering of Christian physicians, Collins suggested that evolution might have been God's elegant plan for creating humankind. Some of the attendees angrily walked out. On questions of how nature works, Collins, like Charles Townes and virtually all scientists of faith, unhesitatingly sides with science. Why then, at the late age of twenty-nine, had Francis Collins become a Christian?

THE CONVERSION ARGUMENT

In the final chapter of his book, Collins summarizes the basis for his religious conversion. It comes down to two points:

- *The anthropic principle:* nature's laws were designed to support life.

- *The moral law*: humans know the difference between right and wrong.

We discussed the anthropic principle at length earlier in this chapter. There is no denying that changes in fundamental constants such as the gravitational constant could make life as we know it impossible. All that tells us is that we don't yet understand why nature's laws are the way they are. Naturalism advises us to be patient. The limits of our understanding are marked with chalk, and will in time be erased by the advance of science. As the frontiers of science advance, seemingly unfathomable mysteries that were once seen as proof of God's existence turn out to be the inevitable consequence of more fundamental laws. Will we ever get to a "final theory" that explains everything and can, as Nobel Prize-winner Leon Lederman put it, "be written on a T-shirt"? Perhaps we never will, but what a magnificent quest.

Even if you accept the anthropic principle as evidence of a creator, it only raises additional questions. The most obvious question is "who created the creator?" And if I try to get around that by arguing that God has always existed, I'm confronted by the next question: "Why the Christian God?" Why not make up a new God? There have been thousands of gods throughout history. What special insight did the authors of the Bible have that leads much of the Western world, thousands of years later, to continue following their god? Even if you see the anthropic principle as implying the existence of a creator, it tells us nothing about that creator except perhaps that he wanted there to be life. The rest is all guesswork and merely tells us what our ancestors wanted their god to be like. The God of the Christian Bible is the God most familiar to the Western world. Unfortunately, this God comes with a lot of baggage including a bunch of preposterous myths. We will examine some of those myths in the following chapters.

Collins' second point, that there is a "moral law," identifies an important research question. The observation that humans have an innate sense of right and wrong goes back thousands of years. The task of science is to understand why. In the two years since Collins called the moral law "the strongest signpost to God," the challenge has been taken up by scientists using some of the latest tools of science.

In chapter 11 we will return to the moral law and its implications for the modern world. But before we can talk about the way *Homo sapiens* should be, there is much to be learned about the way we are and how we got to be that way, beginning with Charles Darwin's theory of evolution by natural selection.

CHAPTER TWO

THE SECRET OF LIFE

*In which Darwin's theory of evolution
by natural selection survives*

Sarah Tishkoff, a young molecular anthropologist at the University of Maryland, believed the out-of-Africa migration of *Homo sapiens* could be tracked by looking for their footprints in the DNA of living humans. It was such a great idea that with funding from a variety of sources, she soon found herself heading an international team of geneticists collecting and analyzing blood samples from populations around the world.

She must also have an adventurous streak. She covered Africa, where modern humans are thought to have originated. It meant driving a Land Rover over hundreds of miles of primitive roads through remote areas with only an interpreter and an assistant. Blood samples had to be centrifuged to remove the perishable red cells using the battery of the Land Rover as power. This reduced the samples to hard, white pellets for analysis back in the United States. Her laptop was powered with a solar panel. Many nights were spent in a tent with animal noises in the background. And always there was concern about political unrest.

Although *Homo sapiens* is thought to have originated in East Africa, the fossil trail is faint. The discovery in 2003 of a single skull in Ethiopia dating back some 160,000 years was major news. Discovered by Tim White and his team from the University of California, Berkeley, it was the oldest known fossil of a modern human, and the strongest evidence yet that *Homo sapiens* did indeed come out of Africa. Over time, our ancestors migrated northward through Egypt and the Middle East, around the Mediterranean, and eventually to northern Europe.

The recent mapping of the human genome provides a new tool for following that ancient trail. Northern Europeans and East Africans might look rather different today, but that's only skin deep. They share an unusual characteristic: they can consume milk into adulthood. Most people on our planet can't. The boy whose skull was found in Ethiopia couldn't. Adult tolerance of lactose wasn't part of the original design of *Homo sapiens*. The gene that produces lactase, the enzyme needed to digest lactose, normally turns off before age four. This forces weaning, freeing the mother to nurse more babies—and babies are what the survival of species is all about.

For most of our 160,000-year history, our *Homo sapiens* ancestors were hunter-gatherers. Lactose tolerance would have offered no advantage. Ancient cave paintings found in the lower Sahara show cattle being herded, but by that time *Homo sapiens* had been around for maybe 150,000 years. Some tribes had discovered that by herding cattle, they could free themselves from the uncertainty of hunting. Domestication of cattle changed everything. In addition to providing meat, it made cow's milk abundant. Lactose, the sugar found in milk, is a major nutrient for babies and adults who can digest it.

Natural selection did its thing. Occasionally, people would have a mutation that kept the lactase gene from turning off. Such a mutation would have offered no advantage to a hunter-gatherer, but for a herder the huge survival advantage of having a source of high-quality protein, especially in lean periods, assured the rapid spread of the mutation. The dairy industry wasn't far behind.

Tishkoff was particularly interested in the milk-tolerance gene. The procedure was to take blood samples from women, measure their glucose levels with a simple tester like those used by diabetics, and then give them milk to drink. An hour later, she would check their glucose levels again. If their glucose levels were up, it meant they had digested the lactose.

There were surprises. When she returned to her lab at Maryland and tested the DNA in the blood samples, she found that the Africans who were lactose tolerant did not have the mutation that conferred lactose tolerance on Northern Europeans. There turned out to be four distinct mutations that conferred lactose tolerance on various African tribes.

It was a stunning confirmation of the power of evolution to meet an important need by random mutations. There are many languages and cultures in East Africa that mix surprisingly little, leading Tishkoff to believe there are additional mutations that have not yet been discovered that have conferred lactose tolerance on other African tribes.

Those who deny the evidence of evolution often lay down a challenge: if evolution is real, why aren't we evolving? The answer is, we are. Evolution tends to be most rapid among isolated populations adapting to unique local environments, and there are few isolated populations left. Evolution is slowed by gene mixing among populations living in different environments— and humans are notorious for sleeping around. However, an adaptation that benefits people in all environments, such as resistance to the 1918 influenza virus, can spread around the world very rapidly thanks to modern transportation.

Because it provides such significant health advantages, lactose tolerance is beginning to show up even in the Far East, where it had been unseen. In a short period of time, by evolutionary standards, the entire world will be lactose tolerant. If anyone is looking for a marker, an ice cream parlor has reportedly opened in Beijing.

Homo sapiens is still evolving, with an enormous gene pool in the world and modern transportation to ensure rapid gene mixing. Changes in the human genome will be limited to those that offer a clear advantage to the entire population, such as lactose tolerance and resistance to new strains of the flu virus. In light of the overwhelming evidence of evolution that has developed since the discovery of the structure of DNA, scientists find it difficult to believe that anyone still denies the reality of evolution—but as we will see, some do.

WHAT DEBATE?

In an interview with Texas reporters on August 1, 2005, President George W. Bush called for "intelligent design" to be taught in science class alongside evolution as competing theories. "I feel like both sides ought to be properly taught," he said, "so people can understand what the debate is about."

But there is no debate, not within the science community. Had the president of the United States just declared war on science? Even John Marburger, head of the White House Office of Science and Technology Policy, told The *New York Times* that the President had been "misunderstood." A physicist and former director of Brookhaven National Laboratories, Marburger described evolution as "the cornerstone of modern biology." By contrast, he said, "intelligent design is not a scientific concept." Marburger was exactly right, but he needed to be telling this to President Bush, not to the *New York Times*. Teaching intelligent design in a biology class would be like teaching astrology to a class in astronomy.

The concept of evolution in biology did not originate with Darwin. In particular, Jean-Baptiste Lamarck had proposed a theory of evolution half a century before Darwin. What differed in Lamarckian evolution was not the concept of a progression of life forms, but the mechanism by which change occurs. Lamarck proposed that offspring must inherit characteristics acquired during the lifetime of the parents, such as the musculature of a trained athlete. It was a brilliant conjecture that sought to explain the changes that take place in species to adapt to new environments. It was the right idea, but the wrong mechanism.

To gain acceptance, new scientific theories must be confirmed by independent testing, and to ensure that scientists are not misled by faulty tests, they must be conducted openly. Even then, findings are conditional. Scientists will revisit a theory whenever new data, or a better way of analyzing the data, become available. Lamarckian evolution simply did not agree with available evidence.

When the famous biologist Thomas Huxley first heard Darwin explain his theory, he reportedly slapped his forehead and exclaimed, "Now why didn't I think of that?" In retrospect the idea seemed obvious. Moreover, Huxley realized at once that a huge amount of confirming evidence already existed. Even the most skeptical scientists soon recognized what a powerful idea it is.

Today, evolution by natural selection is the organizing principle that underlies the entire field of biology. Thousands upon thousands of articles based on Darwinian evolution have been published in peer-reviewed scientific journals. The authors include many of the world's leading scientists. By one count, thirty-eight of the last fifty Nobel prizes in physiology and medicine were directly related to evolution.

Darwin's theory had freed the human mind from the shackles of tradition. In terms of the number of seemingly unrelated pieces of information it tied together, evolution by natural selection is the most successful scientific theory ever conceived. Moreover, it opened up a way of thinking about the universe that goes far beyond biology. It was the beginning of naturalism.

Living organisms had heretofore been considered far too complex to be the product of purely natural processes, and every new discovery revealed additional layers of complexity. They seemed to require a supernatural intelligence—an intelligent design. Then, along comes this new theory of evolution by natural selection that seemed to say that the almost unimaginable complexity of living things is simply the result of blind natural forces acting over a very long time.

Where had the belief in a creator come from in the first place? Is it possible, scientists began to ask, that the whole concept of a creator is unnecessary?

THE CREATION MYTH

People have always longed to know why there is a world, and why the world is the way it is, but for most of history such knowledge was hopelessly beyond human reach. Storytellers sat around the fire spinning imaginative tales to account for the world and the unseen forces that control our lives. Creation myths sought to explain where humans came from. The most compelling of these stories were passed on to subsequent generations. With every retelling and every embellishment, these myths must have seemed more natural—even obvious. For 160,000 years, superstition held *Homo sapiens* captive.

Today, every culture still has a central creation myth. Western culture is dominated by three great religions, Judaism, Christianity, and Islam, that share a common creation myth: the Genesis story of Adam and Eve. Genesis was translated from ancient Hebrew texts written more than three thousand years ago, parts of which, including the great flood, were borrowed from *Gilgamesh*, a Sumerian epic that is the oldest known written story, composed five thousand years ago. Nevertheless, religious fundamentalists believe the biblical scriptures, including the Genesis account of creation, to be the inerrant, divinely inspired word of God and must therefore be interpreted literally. Since it's the literal truth, they argue, it should be taught to their children in biology class.

The intelligent-design theory that the President called for teaching alongside evolution in science class is not Genesis. In an effort to get around the Establishment Clause of the First Amendment, intelligent design avoids any mention of "creation" or "God," focusing instead on the extreme complexity of human physiology, which it argues could not have happened by chance. Proponents hoped this would be seen as proof that an unidentified intelligence was involved in the design of living things. Intelligent design does not involve any new scientific findings, nor has it been used in a single research paper in a peer-reviewed scientific journal. Intelligent design is merely a strategy, a tactic in a holy war fought to put God back in the classroom—and keep Darwin out.

The great irony is that the war is over a theory that neither side believes—certainly not the scientists, who overwhelmingly accept Darwinian evolution, but not even the Christian fundamentalists, who would have preferred the story of Adam and Eve. As in all wars, the strategy is just to win. As we will see, some committed Christians even volunteered to serve behind enemy lines as double agents, earning a PhD in biology to be more effective in the war against Darwinism—an extreme example of what has been called "sacred dishonesty."

PATTERNS

Our ability to make sense of the world begins with the marvelous ability of the human brain to pick out patterns in the information collected by our senses. Recognizing familiar patterns in unfamiliar situations is the beginning of reasoning by analogy, and therefore of abstract thought. Our savage ancestors, living as hunter-gatherers in a Pleistocene wilderness, must have been very good at figuring out the behavior patterns of the animals they hunted for food, as well as those that hunted them for food. Just to find grubs, you must know to turn the log over.

Remarkably, it would turn out that the brain that was good at finding grubs and avoiding saber-toothed tigers could also recognize more abstract patterns in language and mathematics. Even more remarkable is the amount of pleasure patterns give us. Whether in music, poetry, or physics, pattern recognition is at the heart of all aesthetic enjoyment.

As we become more sophisticated in whatever it is we do, we learn to recognize ever-more subtle patterns. It's a thin line, however, between recognizing subtle patterns and apophenia: seeing patterns where none exist. A form of schizophrenia, apophenia is often associated with brilliance, like that of John Nash, portrayed in the movie *A Beautiful Mind*. Nash would eventually be awarded the Bank of Sweden Prize in Economic Sciences in Honor of Alfred Nobel for his brilliant work in game theory, but as the movie shows, his tendency to apophenia at times led him dangerously astray.

It is should be noted that although Nash is almost always referred to as a "Nobel Laureate," the Bank of Sweden Prize was not actually included in Alfred Nobel's will. Nevertheless, the Bank of Sweden Prize deliberately mimics the Nobel pattern and it is usually referred to as simply the Nobel Prize in Economics.

Humans all seem to be on the verge of apophenia. The brain that is able to link the tides to the phases of the moon may also see in the passage of a comet an omen of victory in battle, or perhaps link a distant supernova to the birth of a god. A strategy is needed to tell which patterns are significant, and which are merely a coincidence. It took 160,000 years before such a strategy was found. We call it science.

THE BIRTH OF SCIENCE

On the 28th of May, 585 BC, there was a solar eclipse. The narrow swath of totality passed over the Greek island of Mellitus. People have always been awed and frightened by eclipses, though few of us will be so fortunate as to personally witness a total eclipse of the Sun. Every culture had its own eclipse myth, perhaps involving an evil monster devouring the Sun. It was up to the priests or shamans to devise a ceremony or incantation that would drive the monster off. They were good at their job—the Sun always emerged unscathed. The priests no doubt claimed full credit for saving the world from catastrophe.

What distinguished the eclipse of 585 BC from every previous eclipse of the Sun by the Moon was that it had been predicted. Thales of Mellitus, or so it is claimed, calculated that the Moon would pass between the Sun and the Earth on that day, temporarily blocking the Sun's light. Many science historians are doubtful that Thales could have done so because the orbit of the Moon is tilted about five degrees with respect to the orbit of the Earth around the Sun, and the shadow of the Moon usually misses Earth completely. Moreover, the dark inner shadow of the Moon responsible for totality sweeps over a narrow path on the Earth's surface that is only about a hundred miles wide. This swath passes over a particular location on Earth only once every 375 years.

Thales may have "predicted" the eclipse in 585 BC after it happened, which is not unusual in ancient historical accounts. In any case, Thales understood what had happened and made use of the event to state the law of cause and effect, perhaps the most brilliant insight of all time: for every physical effect there is a physical cause. Causality abolishes superstition.

But the world wasn't looking for a cause. People thought they already knew what caused eclipses. Eclipses were not thought of as "natural" events; they were believed to be supernatural— almost everything was. God made the Sun rise, sent storms, shook the Earth, and sometimes God blotted out the Sun. Who are we mortals to question why God would do these things? The most humans could hope to do was to placate an angry God with offerings and flattery.

We have little direct evidence of what people thought before the invention of writing, which was about five thousand years ago. Based on artifacts and cave drawings, however, archeologists conclude that early humans probably practiced magic, as primitive tribes still do today. Sometimes it worked, sometimes it didn't. The practical problem for shamans, therefore, was to fiddle with the ceremonies and incantations to invent more reliable magic. They also advised people to avoid anything that might offend the spirits—and of course, leave generous offerings on the altar.

Not much has changed; that's basically where we are today. Polls consistently show that about 90% of the U.S. population firmly believes in an all-powerful Creator/God, and most pray to that God, many as often as five times a day. Sometimes, as with restoring the Sun during an eclipse, it works, sometimes it doesn't.

Richard Feynman, perhaps the most admired physicist of our time, described science as "what we have learned about how not to fool ourselves." Thales was a teacher, not a magician. He did not claim to control the eclipse, only to explain it. Mysteries are the stuff of shamans and holy men. Scientists hate mysteries. They make their findings, including the details of how they were obtained, available to the scrutiny of everyone. If someone comes up with more accurate measurements or a better analysis of the data, the textbooks are rewritten.

There are no final answers. It sounds like a prescription for chaos, and when scientists announce a new explanation, it's often frustrating to nonscientists, who ask why scientists can't make up their minds. The alternative, however, is dogma. Openness sets science apart from all other ways of knowing. Anything else is superstition.

Science has thrown open the book of nature. On its pages we are finding, if not a simple world, at least an orderly world: a world in which everything from the birth of stars to falling in love is governed by the same natural laws. Much of the book of nature remains to be read, but already *Homo sapiens* has unraveled the genetic code, sent robots to explore distant planets, and put all of the world's knowledge at the fingertips of ordinary people. Life expectancy has doubled, hunger has been reduced to a political problem, machines have taken over the mind-numbing toil that had been the lot of common folk, and many of the dreaded diseases that once tormented our species can now be cured or even eradicated from the earth.

During the seventeenth and eighteenth centuries, in the period called the Enlightenment, educated people thought the most important benefit of science would be to free the world

from superstition. Unfortunately, that did not happen. Even as
people embrace the gifts of science, they cling to ancient superstitions learned at their mother's knee. The more implausible
the belief, the more virtuous it is deemed to persist in it. How
are we to account for the persistence of superstition in this age
of science?

TURNING ON THE LIGHT

When I was boy of ten, I had a dog of uncertain ancestry named
Buster. A large dog, Buster slept in the barn, and I was forbidden to bring him into the house. One cold night, however, I
smuggled Buster into my room. As I clicked on the light in my
room I wondered what Buster must be thinking. Buster must
see me as very powerful, I thought. Controlling light is the sort
of thing gods do. If Buster was impressed, however, he managed to hide it. Dogs, I came to realize, don't puzzle over how
things work. But neither, it seems, do many people.

People who are quick to make use of the Global Positioning
System (GPS), or BlackBerrys, or beta-blockers, or any of the
other wonders of modern technology, often exhibit no more
interest in how such things might work than Buster did in how
I controlled light. If some know-it-all scientist insists on trying to explain these things, people understandably become im-
patient. The explanations, after all, often fall outside the range
of space and time in which people live their lives: the distance
of their daily commute, for example, or the brief span of
human life.

Van Leeuwenhoek's microscope and Galileo's telescope took
scientists into the realms of the very small and the very distant.
With our instruments we obtain images of distant galaxies and
probe the nucleus of atoms, measure the distance between stars
and the size of an atom. But we can't go there. We can learn
about the past from relics and fossils, but we can't go there either. As for the future, we will get there all too soon. The only

certainty is that we will wish for more time to explore these other realms than we will be given.

Homo sapiens is a comparatively recent addition to the animal family. Anthropologists have unearthed remains of our species that are 160,000 years old, and yet all of written history goes back only 5,000 years. How much has *Homo sapiens* changed in 160,000 years?

To borrow from the movie *Jurassic Park*, suppose a mosquito gorged on the blood of one of our *Homo sapiens* ancestors 160,000 years ago, and then became entrapped in amber, providing modern scientists with ancient human DNA. And further suppose that this ancient DNA is used to clone a human, who is then raised from infancy in today's society. What if it has already happened and a Pleistocene clone is enrolled in my physics class? Could I pick out the Pleistocene clone from the rest of the class? Probably not—individual variations are too great. My students don't look alike or think alike. God knows there's room for improvement, but I'm fond of them all.

Some recent evidence purports to show that there may have been a few subtle changes in the brain of *Homo sapiens* over tens of thousands of years, probably associated with language, and as we saw, lactose tolerance is spreading through the population. The driving force of evolution is change in the environment. Why then haven't humans evolved to cope with a world that little resembles the world that our Pleistocene ancestors lived in?

Change is most rapid when a species is isolated in a particular environment, such as the finches Darwin encountered in the Galapagos Archipelago. Unable to fly from island to island, populations of Galapagos finches on each island were isolated unless carried by storm winds. Over time finches on each island developed distinctive beaks according to the kinds of seeds that were most abundant.

Humans, for better or worse, are notorious for spreading their genes outside their own tribe. The mixing of human genes among populations that cope with very different environments has the effect of suppressing evolution.

Homo sapiens today struggles to cope in a world of jet travel and wireless communication while saddled with almost stagnant genes selected for life as hunter-gathers in a Pleistocene wilderness. It's not as dire as that makes it sound. We make our own habitat, and we make it to suit the genes we have. There is room for improvement.

EVOLUTION IN THE CLASSROOM

We are living in an era of transition from the traditional worldview of the great religions to a modern worldview based on naturalism. The transition was accelerated by Charles Darwin. To protect their children from this heretical idea, creationists seek to prevent evolution from being taught in public schools. Most people, including some scientists, manage to straddle religious and scientific worldviews, choosing items from both menus. While educated people may accept the fact that the laws of nature govern the behavior of material bodies, they are often reluctant to believe that the dreams and emotions that stir within themselves can be reduced to the laws of physics.

The religious right has exploited this ambivalence to pass laws restricting the teaching of evolution in a number of states, even though the First Amendment to the U.S. Constitution prohibits the passage of any law that would serve to establish a state religion.

The first court test of such a law was the famous 1925 Scopes Trial in Dayton, Tennessee, also called the "monkey trial." John Scopes was convicted of violating the Butler Act, passed by the Tennessee General Assembly just a few months earlier, which barred the teaching of evolution. A young high school science teacher, Scopes had been put up to it by a group of local citizens who assumed he would be found guilty, but who hoped the case could be appealed to the federal courts, where it would be found unconstitutional.

They were only half right. It was a healthy airing of the evolution controversy, with high-profile public figures coming in on both sides of the issue, attracting intense media coverage. As expected, Scopes was found guilty and paid a $100 fine, setting the stage for an appeal in federal court. However, Scopes's conviction was reversed on a technicality later that year, without the constitutionality of the Butler Act ever being tested in a higher court.

Thirty years later the Scopes trial was dramatized in a Broadway play *Inherit the Wind* that has been hailed as one of the great American plays of the twentieth century, and in 1960 a Hollywood version became the world's first in-flight movie when TWA featured it to lure first-class passengers.

The Scopes trial may have given an increasingly multicultural nation its first hard look at the conflict between faith and science, but from a legal standpoint the failure of the Scopes case to be tested in federal court was a serious setback for science.

It would be forty-three years after the Scopes "monkey trial" before the constitutionality of laws prohibiting the teaching of evolution in public schools would at last be examined by the U.S. Supreme Court.

That left the way open for fundamentalists in Arkansas to pass their own 1928 law prohibiting any public school or university from teaching "the theory or doctrine that mankind ascended or descended from a lower order of animals" and from using any textbook that taught the same. The law remained in effect for four decades without anyone being prosecuted for violating it.

A Little Rock high school teacher, Susan Epperson, volunteered to serve as the Arkansas Scopes. Rather than have her deliberately violate the law as John Scopes had done, lawyers for the Arkansas Educational Association asked her to request a declaratory judgment on the law. As expected, state courts upheld the law, and the case was appealed to the U.S. Supreme Court.

In 1968, the U.S. Supreme Court in *Epperson v. Arkansas* invalidated the Arkansas statute, holding that it violated the Establishment Clause of the First Amendment. Ironically, the general assembly in Tennessee, anticipating the outcome, had revoked the Butler Act just a few months earlier. Creationism has been in full retreat ever since, with creationists defending one fallback position after another.

As every teacher knows, many lessons are learned only by repetition. A few years after the defeat of the Arkansas law, Louisiana passed its own equal-treatment law, the 1987 Creationism Act. It prohibited the teaching of evolution in Louisiana schools unless it was accompanied by instruction in "creation science." By now you know the pattern. Later that same year, in *Edwards v. Aguillard*, the U.S. Supreme Court found that, by advancing the belief that a supernatural being had created humankind, the Louisiana Creationism Act impermissibly endorsed religion.

It began to dawn on the creationists that they needed a new strategy.

DESIGNING A NEW STRATEGY

While all this was going on in the courts, Phillip Johnson, a distinguished law professor at the University of California, Berkeley, was in the midst of a personal crisis. A former law clerk for liberal-leaning Chief Justice Earl Warren, Johnson had initially opposed the Vietnam War. Offended by the increasingly rowdy antiwar movement at Berkeley, however, Johnson began turning to the right, even as his artist wife became an ardent feminist and turned left. Devastated by the collapse of his marriage, Phillip Johnson turned to Jesus Christ.

From a Christian perspective, Johnson felt he had squandered his intellectual talents on matters of little significance.

Searching for a purpose, he traveled to London in 1987 on sabbatical. In a 2005 interview with Michael Powell of the *Washington Post*, Johnson recalled picking up a copy of *The Blind Watchmaker* in a London bookstore. A 1986 bestseller by Oxford professor Richard Dawkins, the title gently mocks the lovely metaphor with which William Paley opened his 1802 book, *Natural Theology*. On finding a watch and a stone lying in a field, a reasonable person would recognize at once that the watch, unlike the stone, has been constructed for some well-defined purpose. Paley observes that every indication of contrivance, every manifestation of design, which existed in the watch, exists in greater degree in the works of nature. The watch must therefore have a maker, Paley reasons—and living things must have a designer.

Dawkins writes in the beginning pages of *The Blind Watchmaker* that "Paley's argument is made with passionate sincerity and is informed by the best biological scholarship of his day, but it is wrong, gloriously and utterly wrong." The rest of the book consists of Dawkins's eloquent and fascinating description of how natural selection, operating over countless generations, shaped all living things. He added the subtitle: Why the evidence of evolution reveals a universe without design.

Johnson had found his purpose. He would defeat the scientific materialism of Dawkins and replace it with a theistic understanding that nature and humans are both creations of God. By the time he left London, Johnson had drafted his response to *The Blind Watchmaker*.

THE GOD OF THE GAPS

Published in 1991, Johnson's book, *Darwin on Trial*, was more a prosecutor's brief than a scientific treatise. While offering no evidence for divine creation other than the obvious complexity of life, Johnson focused on the "gaps" in the chain of evidence for evolution. This comes perilously close to the argument that the domain of God consists of those things science cannot explain. Such a God is often referred to as the "God of the gaps." His domain must inevitably shrink as scientific knowledge expands.

The gaps often refer to the fossil record. In 1859, when Darwin wrote *On the Origin of Species*, it was all gaps. Collecting fossils was little more than a hobby among the well-to-do. Darwin himself was an avid fossil collector. Collecting fossils became the science of paleontology only after Darwin's theory gave it organization. Considering the almost unimaginable time span it covers, paleontologists find it remarkable that the fossil record is as complete as it is. The standard joke among paleontologists is that every time the fossil of a "missing link" is discovered, it adds another gap—where there was one gap there are now two, one on either side of the new fossil link.

Although proponents of intelligent design see every fossil gap as unbridgeable, new fossils keep turning up. Even as I write these words, fossils of a 375-million year-old fish have been found in the Canadian Arctic, six hundred miles from the North Pole. It was a fish with a swivel head, a wrist, and an elbow. It appears to be a perfect candidate for an intermediate species between sea and land-dwelling animals. The excitement of its discovery is captured by Neil Shubin in *Your Inner Fish*.

There was, however, a much more serious gap in Darwin's theory. Evolution by natural selection requires some mechanism for passing on characteristics from parents to offspring. Darwin saw at once that it could not just be a blending of characteristics from the parents. In that case, a beneficial change would be diluted with each succeeding generation. Darwin speculated that there had to be discrete units of inheritance that might come from either parent. It was Darwin's genius to predicate his monumental theory on the existence of these unknown units of inheritance, confident that they would be found.

What Darwin didn't know was that in Moravia at that time an Augustinian monk named Gregor Mendel was experimenting with the inheritance of plant characteristics. His work would later form the basis of the modern field of genetics, and the units of inheritance would be called "genes." But Mendel's work received little attention until long after both he and Darwin were dead.

FILLING IN THE GAPS

It was almost a hundred years after Darwin wrote *Origin of Species* that James Watson and Francis Crick left the Cavendish Laboratory at Cambridge on Saturday, February 28, 1953, knowing they had just worked out the structure of the DNA molecule, which by then was recognized as the repository of genetic information. They stopped by the Eagle, a pub they frequented near the lab. Crick raised his glass and to all in earshot announced, "We have discovered the secret of life."

And they had. They had unraveled the structure of the molecule that determines heredity, the blueprint of every living thing on earth. The world was forever changed. Not only had they confirmed Charles Darwin's conjecture about the units of inheritance responsible for evolution, they had provided the world with the means to quantify the evolutionary relationship between all living things. If the evidence for evolution had been persuasive before, it was now irrefutable.

Watson and Crick would share the 1962 Nobel Prize for determining the double-helix structure of DNA. Watson would later relate the story in a best-selling 1968 book, *The Double Helix*. He would go on to become director of the Cold Spring Harbor Laboratory on Long Island, and build it into one of the world's leading research institutions in molecular biology. Reaping the full benefits for humanity of unraveling the mystery of DNA, however, would require mapping the entire human genome consisting of 24 chromosomes, with some 3 billion DNA base pairs containing perhaps 25,000 genes.

It was a daunting prospect, impossible in 1968, but by 1988 it began to seem possible. Recent advances in computers and gene-sequencing techniques had made it possible to map the human genome, but it would be a massive project. Who better to head the project than James Watson?

Soon after the Human Genome Project got underway, however, J. Craig Venter, who was at that time an obscure geneticist, brashly announced that the government project might as well close down because his private company would finish the job first. Venter founded The Institute for Genomic Research and declared that using improved equipment he could do the job by 2001—three years before Watson expected to complete the job.

THE NAKED GENETICIST

Craig Venter was the son of an alcoholic father who was excommunicated from the Mormon Church. He grew up a working-class neighborhood near Half Moon Bay, California, showing little promise in high school for anything except surfing. He enlisted in the navy during the Vietnam War, as those of limited means are often forced to do. The navy saw something else in him, training him to become a medical corpsman, and shipping him off to the Da Nang hospital in Vietnam. The horror of that experience left him determined to know more about medical science. After his tour in the navy, Venter sailed through the University of California, San Diego, earning a PhD in physiology. Initially recruited by NIH as the Human Genome Project was getting underway, Venter came up with a faster method of sequencing and left NIH to found Celera, a company that sought to patent its genomic information.

Watson, angered that Venter had been allowed to turn the Human Genome Project into a drag race, was fiercely opposed to patenting genetic information. Bernadine Healy, the NIH director, sided with Venter on the issue of patenting genomes, forcing Watson to resign as head of the Human Genome Project in 2002. He returned to Cold Spring Harbor Laboratory, where he became president. In a final sad chapter in his distinguished career, Watson, who had a habit of sometimes thinking out loud, was quoted in a London newspaper as suggesting that black Africans might be less intelligent than Europeans. No one who knows James Watson believes he meant it the way it came out, but words cannot be unspoken.

Francis Collins, the NIH geneticist we met in chapter 1, was named to replace Watson as head of the academic consortium that made up the Human Genome Project. A year later the Human Genome Project announced that it had successfully decoded the entire genome. There were still a few gaps, however, and only the male haploid genome had been decoded. Moreover, it was made up of pieces from people of different racial and ethnic backgrounds. It would be better, the experts thought, to have the diploid genome of a single person.

The other runner in the race, meanwhile, just kept running. Craig Venter snorted that the consortium had stopped halfway to the finish line. In 2007, Venter released the full diploid genome of a single person—himself. The experts seem to agree that Venter's genome is better.

That's not to say he has better genes. Craig Venter now stands naked before the world, his genes exposed to public view. He has genes linked to Alzheimer's, alcoholism, obesity, antisocial behavior, tobacco addiction, substance abuse, and wet earwax. If there's a gene for vanity, he's probably got that too. Having those genes does not mean he has those conditions. They take more than a single gene to be expressed. It is easy to see why Privacy advocates have concerns about the new technology. But by using his own genome, Venter had avoided all sorts of entanglements—and satisfied his vanity.

The point of all this is that science has moved far beyond any question of the reality of evolution. To argue against Darwinism now would be like claiming the New World does not exist because it doesn't show up on maps drawn before the voyage of Columbus. It's past time for the world to move on, but of course it hasn't.

DESIGNING INTELLIGENT DESIGN

Not everyone gets it. In a 2005 interview with Michael Powell of the *Washington Post*, Phillip Johnson, the lawyer turned creationist, described his reaction to Darwinian evolution: "I realized that if the pure Darwinist account was accurate and life is all about an undirected material process, then Christian metaphysics and religious belief are fantasy. Here was a chance to make a great contribution."

It looked more like the making of a perfect storm. Phillip Johnson had not picked an easy opponent. Dawkins's 1976 book, *The Selfish Gene*, was a huge contribution to the understanding of evolution by scientists. It had vaulted him to a rank among the leaders in the challenging field of evolutionary biology. Remarkably, it had at the same time, like Watson's *Double Helix*, become a best seller among the general public. *The Selfish Gene* is the book Charles Darwin would have written if Watson and Crick had discovered the structure of DNA a century earlier.

Phillip Johnson and Richard Dawkins are antimatter conjugates. They look at the same evidence, but their brains register inverted images. Should they ever come in contact, it would not surprise me if like a positron and an electron, they vanish in a burst of energy.

Even though he is not a scientist, Johnson is recognized as the father of the intelligent design movement. He saw that getting beyond the Establishment Clause of the First Amendment called for a scientific argument—or at least a scientific-sounding argument. He steeped himself in the scientific literature on evolution and soon began to imagine that he understood the science more clearly than did the scientists. It is not the logic of evolution that concerned Johnson, however, so much as the self-indulgent behavior he associated with people who don't believe they are accountable to God to for their actions. There is, as we will discuss more fully in a later chapter, no evidence at all that the faithful lead more morally disciplined lives than the skeptics. The false conviction that they do is the historical justification for state-imposed religion—the very thing the Establishment Clause of the First Amendment was intended to prevent.

Johnson's 1991 book, *Darwin on Trial*, did not exactly foment a revolution, but it did mark the founding of the intelligent design movement. For the next step he would need an organization and resources. He would also need some scientific cover, but there were no scientists sympathetic to intelligent design—or at least no scientists of any stature. Biologists and paleontologists were not interested in the views of a law professor who had no background in science and yet proposed to challenge the basic tenet of modern biology. The best he could come up with was Stephen Meyer, a graduate student in the philosophy of science at Cambridge whom he had met on his London sabbatical—not really a scientist, but maybe close enough.

After graduating from Cambridge, Meyer taught philosophy at a couple of small Christian colleges. In 1990, he hooked up with an out-of-office politician named Bruce Chapman to form the Discovery Institute in Seattle, Washington, a nonprofit educational foundation and think tank based on the Christian apologetics of C. S. Lewis and opposed to "materialism."

The basic assumption of modern science, and the dominant worldview of our time, is naturalism, which holds that whatever happens in the world can be explained by the laws of nature. Simply stated, there is no magic. The Discovery Institute, however, avoids ever using the word "naturalism," using instead the term "scientific materialism." Why the change? "Natural" carries a positive connotation. While "materialism" can mean the same thing as "naturalism," it can also mean an obsessive desire for worldly possessions, giving it a more negative connotation. Words matter. Even the title "Discovery Institute" is chosen to convey an image of scientific research, whereas the organization conducts no research.

Everything seemed to be falling into place just as Phillip Johnson had planned. "Intelligent design," backed by Johnson's teach-the-controversy strategy, had captured the imagination of ultra-conservative donors with very deep pockets, including Howard Ahmanson Jr. and the MacLellan Foundation. The Discovery Institute agreed to create a Center for Science and Culture, devoted solely to promoting intelligent design. Stephen Meyer was appointed as the director and "senior fellow" of the Center, and Phillip Johnson as the "senior advisor."

Johnson laid out a five-year plan. The immediate goal was to win in the court of public opinion, and win they did—for a time. They were winning by following a strict set of rules laid down by Johnson. It's the sort of strategy you might want to follow, but not the sort you would want to advertise:

- Don't get involved in details or arguments over scientific facts.
- Forget about the great flood and the age of the Earth.
- Don't mention the Bible or creation, much less God.
- Keep the focus on the "gaps" in evolution.
- The fallback position is, "Teach the controversy."

It's a strategy of deception, an attempt to divert attention from the scientific emptiness of the intelligent design argument.

INCONVENIENT TRUTHS

Before long, nineteen states were considering legislation to mandate education in intelligent design along with evolution. Intelligent design was all over the news, but it still had not been tested in the courts. A lot needed to be done to get ready for the inevitable day in court.

To carry out Phillip Johnson's strategy, the intelligent design movement needed financial benefactors. Potential benefactors want to know how their money will be spent. They have to be let in on the strategy, increasing the risk of disclosure. The Center for Science and Culture hired a public relations firm to help with the increasing volume of mail. The Center was filled with deeply committed conservative Christians. But the PR firm was not.

In January of 1999, an employee of the firm was given a ten-page document labeled *The Wedge* to copy. It was stamped "TOP SECRET. Curious, he made an extra copy for himself. Within days, the cynical and deceptive *Wedge* was on the Web for the world to see. By 2004, *The Wedge* had become the subject of a scholarly book by two prominent academics. In *Creationism's Trojan Horse*, Barbara Forrest, a philosopher, and Paul Gross, a physiologist, meticulously traced the origins of the intelligent design movement back to its creationist underpinnings.

Secrecy does not belong in a democracy. It may seem that in a dangerous world, even democracies have little choice but to secure certain kinds of information against public disclosure, such as details of weapons systems. Every secret, however, carries with it a heavy cost in corruption and inefficiency, as well as the erosion of ethical principles.

Those in power, of course, love official secrets. It gives them complete control over the release of information. Governments classify as "secret" anything that might be embarrassing to them, and leak information that makes them look good. White House press secretary Scott McClellan once explained that the president does not leak any secrets, since anything he chooses to reveal is declassified automatically.

Democracy's last line of defense may be government insiders who are willing to jeopardize their careers, and even risk going to jail, to reveal embarrassing truths that are hidden behind the shroud of official secrecy. The 1971 leak of the Pentagon Papers by Daniel Ellsberg accelerated the end of the Vietnam War. The leak of the Pentagon's Nuclear Posture Review in 2002 and of the secret CIA-run prisons for suspected terrorists in Eastern Europe in 2006 exposed policies the public would not have condoned. The only certain protection against leaks would be to operate completely in the open. That choice is not often taken.

Private organizations with controversial agendas, such as the Discovery Institute and its Center for Science and Culture, also choose to operate in secrecy; but they are no more successful at it than the government. The leak of *The Wedge* was just the beginning; other inconvenient truths were bound to come out.

ICONS OF DECEPTION

The Center for Science and Culture has recruited dozens of "fellows" to promote its cause. Some are from small Christian colleges, but many hold PhDs from prestigious universities. Jonathon Wells, a senior fellow, is a cell biologist with a PhD from the University of California, Berkeley. In 2000 he wrote *Icons of Evolution: Science or Myth,* or "Why much of what we teach about evolution is wrong." The Discovery Institute trumpeted his appointment as proof of a commitment to "sound science." *Icons of Evolution*, however, was a disaster. It may have been popular with the Kansas School Board, but every scientist who bothered to read it savaged it.

Wells seems particularly incensed by the great American biologist Theodosius Dobzhansky's observation that "nothing in biology makes sense except in the light of evolution." It was actually the title of an article Dobzhansky wrote for *The American Biology Teacher* in 1973, just two years before his death. Every biologist I know agrees completely with Dobzhansky, who was surely the most influential American biologist of his time.

In *Icons of Evolution*, Wells accuses Dobzhansky of "dogmatism," and seems quite unaware of the massive irony of such a charge. Dobzhansky devoted his entire life to resisting dogmatism. In 1927, as his native Russia fell under the spell of the mad biologist Trofim Lysenko, Dobzhansky and his wife immigrated to the United States rather than abide by Lysenko's decrees. Lysenko had been put in charge of Soviet agriculture, and pressured Soviet officials into banning the teaching of

Darwin's theory of evolution by natural selection in favor of Jean-Baptiste Lamarck's earlier mechanism of inheritance of acquired characteristics.

Lamarck proposed his theory to explain the progression of life forms fifty years before Darwin published the *Origin of Species*, but continued to have supporters until late in the twentieth century. Lamarck's theory was a brilliant speculation, but suffered the serious weakness of not agreeing with the evidence. No matter, Lamarkian evolution resonated with Marx's doctrine of dialectic materialism, and Lysenko was given enormous influence over Russian agriculture. The result was widespread starvation due to crop failures, and estrangement of Soviet biology from the explosive progress in the rest of the industrialized world that had been triggered by Darwin's theory. Russian biology has never fully recovered from Lysenko, and it still trails the rest of the industrialized world.

Not only did Wells revise the history of terrestrial life in his book, he revised his personal life history in the preface. Wells writes in the preface that as a graduate student of biology at the University of California, Berkeley, he thought at first that most of what he was taught about evolution was substantially true. Eventually, he writes, he began to realize that textbooks dealing with evolution contain "blatant misrepresentations" which "suggests that Darwinism encourages distortions of the truth."

His recollections are very different in an autobiographical sketch he wrote for the Unification Church. Jonathon Wells is a convert to the Unification Church, founded by the Reverend Sun Myung Moon. From 1976 to 1978 Wells studied at the Unification Theological Seminary. He was flattered when Reverend Moon, whom Wells calls "Father," chose him to enter a PhD program: "Father's words, my studies, and my prayers convinced me that I should devote my life to destroying Darwinism." This hardly sounds like the disillusioned graduate student Wells describes in the preface to his book.

For an obedient disciple of Reverend Sun Myung Moon to accuse Theodosius Dobzhansky of dogmatism is more than ironic.

It is an example of the vice Paul Tillich labeled "sacred dishonesty," in which the facts are revised to support a supposedly worthy conclusion. We will encounter other examples of sacred dishonesty, especially when intelligent design gets its day in court.

COMPARTMENTS

These embarrassments seemed to have little effect on public attitudes toward evolution. According to a Gallup poll taken in the summer of 1999, 45% of adult Americans said they believe in a literal interpretation of the biblical account of creation, and only about one in ten subscribe to a purely scientific interpretation of evolution.

Opinion polls serve an important function in a democracy. We need to have some sense of the public mood on issues, but polls are not elections. What is often difficult to discern in poll numbers is depth of conviction. When people say they believe the Genesis account of creation, what does "believe" mean? How much would these people be willing to wager that Genesis is literally true? Society is not very tolerant of nonbelievers. Even in the anonymity of a poll, many people, if not most, are conditioned by society to avoid saying anything that might offend religious sensitivities. Ways must be found to ask such poll questions in a nonreligious context.

People are, after all, also reluctant to appear ignorant. Since a literal interpretation of Genesis puts the age of the Earth at only about six thousand years, it would be interesting to ask people if they agree with scientists who say dinosaurs lived millions of years ago, omitting any reference to Genesis. In 1999 I suggested such an experiment to a pollster at the *Kansas City Star*, who had been closely following the creationism debate in Kansas. The pollster agreed to the experiment. Based on the Gallup poll results, you would expect no more than half the population to agree with the scientists on the age of dinosaurs.

Instead, 81% said they agreed that dinosaurs lived millions of years ago. Polls such as Gallup are usually represented as highly accurate reflections of what people think, but it's clear from this example that a great deal more thought needs to be given to framing questions in a way that exposes compartmentalization of people's thoughts.

The important lesson for us here is that there is a strong motivation for people to compartmentalize their beliefs. Religious beliefs in particular seem to be held in a separate compartment into which the most obvious common-sense rules that guide us in our daily life never enter. Compartmentalization is essential to understanding how otherwise rational people can hold absurdly superstitious beliefs.

THE SCHOOL BOARD

For such an important responsibility, being on a school board doesn't get you a lot of recognition. Few voters, for example, can name a single member of their local or state school board. That makes school boards a target of opportunity for organized zealots with an agenda.

Religious zealots do not like Charles Darwin. The intelligent design movement counts on that, but there's a pitfall: religious zealots are inclined to go too far. When school boards finally do something truly outrageous, voters wake up and throw them out.

In 2004, a district school board in Dover, Pennsylvania mandated biology teachers to read a statement to their ninth-grade students informing them that: (1) there are gaps in Darwin's theory of evolution; (2) there is an alternative called "intelligent design"; and (3) a book in the school library, *Of Pandas and People*, explains intelligent design.

Individual members of the school board, and many parents, had no interest in the scientific claims made on behalf of intelligent design, nor had they ever looked at *The Wedge*. Like

Phillip Johnson, what they wanted was for students to grow up with Christian values, and to them that meant exposing children to the Holy Bible. But school board members cared nothing about Johnson's carefully thought-out legal strategy. They just didn't want children to be taught one thing on Sunday, only to have them taught another in biology class during the week.

Other parents, concerned that their children were being denied a modern education in biology, filed suit in federal court to block the school board from carrying out the new policy. *Kitzmiller v. Dover Area School District*, usually shortened to just *Kitzmiller*, takes its name from Tammy Kitzmiller, one of the concerned parents. A powerful team of lawyers from the American Civil Liberties Union, Americans United for Separation of Church and State, and the National Center for Science Education was assembled to represent the concerned parents. The conservative Thomas Moore Law Center in Ann Arbor, Michigan, represented the Dover School Board.

It had been expected that lawyers for the well-heeled Discovery Institute would represent the school board. However, although the school board had embraced intelligent design as the latest weapon in the battle against Godlessness, it had paid little attention to Phillip Johnson's carefully crafted "wedge strategy." From the standpoint of the Discovery Institute, the Dover School Board's statement on evolution was a classic example of enthusiastic amateurs going too far. The Discovery Institute sought to distance itself from the Kitzmiller suit, but within its own ranks, two Institute fellows agreed to testify for the school board. A brilliant strategy won't help if discipline can't be maintained among the troops.

It had also been expected that the decision in *Kitzmiller* would be appealed to a higher court, perhaps eventually even to the U.S Supreme Court, thus expanding its legal reach. Concerned that *Kitzmiller* would succeed, but unable to stop the trial, the Discovery Institute sought to play down its significance. They got inadvertent help from the voters. Eight of the nine school board members were up for reelection in the summer of 2005, and the voters defeated all eight.

The new school board members were all elected because they wanted only Darwin's theory of evolution to be taught in biology class. If the decision of the court favored Darwin, it would merely direct the new board to do exactly what its members were pledged to do, so the new board would not appeal. The other side would not appeal because it would be clear that they had not come close, and if appealed to a higher court, the decision would apply more widely.

THE DOVER EFFECT

The Discovery Institute was watching glumly from the sidelines on Monday, September 26, 2005, as *Kitzmiller v. Dover Area School District* got underway in U.S. District Court in Harrisburg, Pennsylvania. Presiding was U.S. District Judge John E. Jones III, appointed to the federal bench in 2002 by George W. Bush. By no stretch an activist judge, both sides agreed that Jones would decide this case on the law.

That afternoon when I joined David and Shaun for our walk beside Northwest Branch, I remarked that the first witness for the plaintiffs in the Dover evolution trial was to be Ken Miller, a highly respected biology professor at Brown University—and a deeply committed Catholic. In his 1999 book, *Finding Darwin's God,* Miller wrote, "To people of faith, what evolution says is that Nature is complete. God fashioned a material world in which truly free, truly independent beings could evolve." Miller is not your typical agnostic academic. Unlike most religious scientists, he does not simply house his beliefs in science and religion in separate compartments. He genuinely seeks to reconcile them. My concern was that the defense lawyers would try to use Miller's religious beliefs to make it appear that he lacked conviction about evolution.

David and Shaun told me not to worry. The Catholic Church, they said, has learned a lot since Galileo. "You'll get no wavering from Catholics on the theory of evolution." Or, as David likes to put it, "The truth is the truth."

As usual, they were right. An attorney for the school board, probing for any hint of softness in Miller's support of Darwin, asked, "Would you agree that Darwin's theory does not represent the absolute truth?" Miller replied without a moment's hesitation: "We do not regard any scientific theory as the absolute truth." He did not need to elaborate. As we discussed in chapter 1, the scientific method requires knowledge to be conditional; if a better explanation comes to light, the textbooks will be rewritten without a backward glance. I could imagine the attorney for the school board mentally crossing out whatever follow-up questions he had prepared. By the end of Miller's testimony, lawyers for the parents must have known that, barring some surprise development, they were going to win.

There were no surprises. Miller had written *Finding Darwin's God* in response to *Darwin's Black Box* by Michael Behe, a little-known biologist at Lehigh University who caught the attention of creationists and evolutionists alike with his 1996 book. It laid out the concept of irreducibly complex molecular systems, such as blood clotting and the immune system. If one of the parts is missing, the system fails. Behe argues that it would be impossible for the parts to evolve separately unless there was a designer managing the project who had a goal in mind. This was the closest thing to a scientific argument for supernatural intervention the creationists could come up with.

Irreducible complexity didn't win many converts. Richard Dawkins dismisses the irreducible-complexity argument as "a pathetic cop-out," and describes Behe as "too lazy to figure out how things work." It became a sort of parlor game among scientists to concoct scenarios by which natural selection could have resulted in Behe's examples of irreducible complexity.

This is the only "science" the defense had going into *Kitzmiller*, and Behe was their lead witness.

His biology was dubious, but there was no doubting his honesty. On cross examination, he acknowledged that the plausibility of intelligent design depends on the extent to which one believes in God.

The trial itself spanned six weeks. Witnesses included members of the school board, scientists, theologians, and others. The evidence they provided was important, but the essence of the trial was captured by the testimony of Ken Miller and Michael Behe. It left little doubt what the outcome would be.

"Our conclusion today," Judge Jones wrote as he summed up his 139-page opinion, "is that it is unconstitutional to teach intelligent design as an alternative to evolution in a public school classroom." His language was scathing.

> Those who disagree with this finding will likely mark it as the product of an activist judge. If so, they will have erred, as this is manifestly not an activist Court. Rather, this case came to us as the result of the activism of an ill-informed faction on a school board, aided by a national public interest law firm eager to find a constitutional test case on intelligent design, who in combination drove the Board to adopt an imprudent and ultimately unconstitutional policy. The breathtaking inanity of the Board's decision is evident when considered against the factual backdrop which has now been fully revealed through this trial.

By this point, the defendants must have been squirming, but the judge still had a final thunderbolt. Because they had violated the plaintiffs' civil rights, he found the board liable for nominal damages as well as the legal costs incurred in vindicating the plaintiffs' constitutional rights.

In other words, school boards everywhere were put on notice that forcing intelligent design or any other form of creationism into the schools could cost them a lot of money. That has cooled the ardor of other school boards that might have been thinking of hopping in bed with the Discovery Institute.

In the wake of the Dover decision, the Ohio Board of Education voted 11–4 to scrap a recently enacted requirement that "critical analysis of evolution" be a part of the biology curriculum. The Discovery Institute had put its full prestige behind Ohio's critical-analysis ploy, proposing it as a model for the entire nation. Instead, intelligent design initiatives were cancelled in California, Indiana, and even Utah.

On Sunday, February 12, 2006, just two months after Judge Jones issued his opinion in *Kitzmiller*, 450 churches around the nation celebrated the birth of Charles Darwin 197 years earlier. The celebrations included special sermons and educational programs that celebrated evolution as God's way of creating man. Perhaps they would have celebrated the occasion anyway, but more likely it was stimulated by media coverage of the Dover trial. The outcome had given courage to rational churchgoers who had been intimidated by a creationist minority.

For many, the Dover trial raised a more troubling question: to what extent had some opponents of evolution, in their zeal to defend the faith, been less than honest?

In the conclusion of his *Kitzmiller* opinion, Judge Jones remarked on how poorly the citizens of the Dover area had been served by members of the school board who voted for the intelligent design policy: "It is ironic that several of these individuals, who so staunchly and proudly touted their religious convictions in public, would time and again lie to cover their tracks and disguise the real purpose behind the intelligent design policy."

Are there other superstitions that persist in spite of clear scientific evidence to the contrary? Alas, many. In the next few chapters, we will take a look at the most common superstitions, starting with prayer.

CHAPTER THREE

MIRACLE AT COLUMBIA

In which both sides pray for victory

President George W. Bush proclaimed a National Day of Prayer and Remembrance to honor the memory of the thousands of victims of the September 11, 2001, terrorist attack and to comfort those who lost loved ones. His proclamation included the gentle promise of Jesus in the Sermon on the Mount, "Blessed are they that mourn, for they shall be comforted." Americans mourned, but there was little comfort. While we grieved for the victims, prayers of thanks were being offered in parts of the world where the terrorists were hailed as martyrs. It was the darkest of all Septembers.

People speak confidently about the power of prayer, but in war both sides pray for victory. The 9/11 terrorist attacks had come at the hands of men of deep faith who prayed to their God that morning for the strength to face certain death so that they might take the lives of total strangers and enter heaven as martyrs. Perhaps they were still muttering prayers with their last breath. Measured by the number of dead and injured, their mission was a spectacular success. Had the God to whom they prayed made it so?

PRAYERS AND PLACEBOS

I would not like to think so. But then, what does any of us know about prayer? According to a 2004 U.S. News & Word Report survey, a majority of Americans say they pray every day, sometimes more than once. They pray mostly for their health or that of loved ones. That makes prayer the most widely practiced of all medical therapies. It is deeply ingrained in our culture. For most of history there was little else anyone could do for the sick, and unlike the bloodletting and purges that were used to treat illness two hundred years ago, prayers at least cause little harm. But what is the evidence that prayer is any more effective than doing nothing?

We recover from most of the injuries and illnesses that afflict us without either prayers or medicine. Like all animals, we have built-in repair mechanisms: broken bones knit, blood clots stop bleeding, damaged nerves regenerate, the immune system mobilizes to destroy invading microorganisms, and so on. Modern medicine can often intervene to assist nature in the healing process, perhaps by administering an antibiotic to fight an infection that threatens to overwhelm the immune system. But if the patient then recovers, how do we know the medicine was responsible?

To obtain FDA approval for a new medicine, it must be convincingly demonstrated in controlled clinical trials that subjects taking the medicine do better on average than those who don't. The revolution of medical science that began in the second half of the twentieth century was made possible by the development of sophisticated statistical methods for evaluating the efficacy of new therapies.

The analysis must take into account the ubiquitous placebo effect, in which patients, expecting their treatment to help, experience at least temporary improvement even though the treatment may have been a sham. The placebo effect is commonly thought of in terms of medically inert substances, such as sugar pills, administered by a trusted physician with assurances that it will help.

Doctors are deliberately exploiting the placebo effect when they prescribe antibiotics for the common cold. Antibiotics have no effect on the cold virus, but recovery will come in a few days anyway, and the placebo effect may make the patient feel better in the meantime. Indeed, patients will often start to feel better before they fill the prescription—or even leave the doctor's office. Although concerns are occasionally raised about the ethics of treating patients with placebos, it's been going on for as long as there have been doctors.

But the doctor's expectations must also be taken into account. A placebo is most likely to work if the doctor genuinely believes it to be a cure and communicates that conviction to the patient. Quack doctors who have a talent for invoking the placebo effect sometimes attract huge followings and wind up on the Oprah Winfrey show.

The randomized placebo-controlled, double-blind trial is perhaps the most important advance in medical research. Neither patient nor the doctor knows whether a treatment is real or a sugar pill. By eliminating even unconscious bias, it makes it possible to determine what works and what doesn't. It used to be referred to as the "mysterious" placebo effect, but it's much less mysterious now, thanks in part to modern brain-imaging technologies. We will look at these remarkable new devices in a later chapter.

But do the clinical trials of new medicines take prayer into account? The *Concise Oxford English Dictionary* that sits on my desk defines prayer as a "request for help addressed to God or another deity." Rather than passively accepting their illness, believers petition an all-powerful and loving God for relief, and are often joined in their petition by friends and family. According to the 2004 U.S. News & World Report survey, those who regularly pray are convinced it helps. Are they fooling themselves?

THE TYRANNY OF THE HYPOTHALAMUS

Perhaps not entirely. Prayer can certainly relieve some of the stress that accompanies injury or illness. Whenever a person experiences pain or fear, the brain initiates the release of hormones into the bloodstream that cause the heart to beat faster, blood pressure, to rise, and respiration to increase. Blood is diverted from the digestive tract to the arms and legs. Even the pupils of the eyes dilate to increase awareness. The body is preparing to fight—or at least to run very fast in the other direction.

But the body is not preparing to heal. If we have suffered an injury, the first priority of our brain is to prevent further injury. Blood is routed primarily to the fighting muscles, not to the site of the injury. This is an emergency—healing will have to wait.

We understand the biochemical mechanism. The hypothalamus, a region at the base of the brain involved in controlling emotions, will instruct the adrenal cortex to release cortisol, a hormone that elevates blood pressure, increases blood glucose levels, and diverts blood from the digestive tract to the brain and limbs. If the hypothalamus continues to call for more cortisol, it will eventually lead to adrenal exhaustion, characterized by extreme fatigue and depression. We simply cannot remain in a heightened state of readiness indefinitely. Even if pain or anxiety persists, the brain must switch to a longer-term strategy.

In a Pleistocene wilderness, a movement in the tall grass betraying the presence of a large animal would have triggered the fight-or-flight response in one of our early *Homo sapiens* ancestors. Indeed, merely visualizing the swaying grass as I composed that line was enough to measurably increase my own pulse rate and alertness—and perhaps yours on reading it. If a fawn had then stepped out of the tall grass instead of the carnivore our ancestor imagined, the stress hormones would have shut off in the period of a single heartbeat. Flight-or-fight is a very ancient response in animals. It was highly developed long before animals emerged from the sea.

Carnivores hiding in the tall grass are not something most of us need to worry about in today's world, but the flight-or-fight response is still very much a part of us. The equivalent of movement in the tall grass might be the shadow cast by a streetlight of someone coming up behind you on a dark street late at night in a dangerous neighborhood.

The body has only a limited number of ways it can respond to anxiety. You might experience much the same physiological response to anxiety before a final exam, or to stage fright before you deliver a speech, or to worry that the tax deduction you just claimed might land you in jail. It's a lousy feeling that hits you right in your blood-deprived stomach. It's perfectly normal, but terribly unpleasant.

PRAYER IN A PROZAC WORLD

The first step to freeing yourself from the tyranny of the hypothalamus is to understand why your brain is making you miserable. Your brain is manipulating you with your own hormones, prodding you to take action to eliminate the cause of the stress. The obvious treatment would be to avoid the tall grass where tigers can hide. But in today's world we have an awful lot of tigers to deal with. Millions of people get relief from anxiety by turning to antidepressants, such as Prozac and Zoloft. They work by boosting levels of serotonin, a brain chemical that constricts blood vessels, countering the effects of stress hormones and elevating your mood.

Although for many people these drugs are a godsend, they don't work for everyone. Dr. Herbert Benson, MD, who heads the Mind-Body Medical Institute and also is connected to Harvard Medical School, recommends a stress-reduction procedure meant to evoke what he calls "the relaxation response." He wrote a best-selling self-help book in 1975 with that title. Even if there is nothing physical that requires healing, the relaxation response can at least cut down on the cortisol, which will get rid of the butterflies in the stomach.

There are obviously a lot of us who suffer from stress in modern society. Dr. Benson's book sold more than 3 million copies. But if you're too stressed to take the time read the book, I can give the secret away in two lines:

- Concentrate on repeating a simple prayer or mantra.
- Ignore the inevitable distractions that come up while you're doing it.

In other words, meditate. It's hardly a new idea. People all over the world have practiced meditation in some form for thousands of years, usually in connection with their religion. Most have done so without ever having read *The Relaxation Response*.

One way to meditate is to pray. You can recite Hail Marys while counting your rosary beads, for example. If you don't have a rosary, chant Buddhist prayers while spinning a prayer wheel, or maybe prostrate yourself on a prayer rug facing east while repeating "God is great." Your respiration will slow, along with your metabolism and pulse rate. However you pray, it can reduce the symptoms of stress and prepare your body for healing. It's no miracle cure, but it can help.

It doesn't seem to matter how or to whom you pray, and it apparently works as well for nonbelievers as for the devout. For that reason, *The Relaxation Response* is offensive to some of the faithful who feel it trivializes prayer. These people aren't looking for self-treatment—they want a God that will intervene on their side and smite their enemies.

To tap into that part of the book market, Benson came out with a second book, *Beyond the Relaxation Response*. It introduces something Benson calls the "faith factor": if you combine the relaxation technique with "your deepest personal beliefs," he explains, it will work even better. He is, in short, prescribing religious faith as a medicine. That book sold well too.

In a recent book, *Blind Faith: The Unholy Alliance of Religion and Medicine*, Richard Sloan, a professor of behavioral medicine at Columbia University, raises serious ethical and practical concerns about doctors prescribing religion for medical problems. If you plan to practice the relaxation response, it would be a good idea to read Sloan's book first.

For relief from intense pain, even atheists grudgingly admit to occasionally succumbing to an impulse to pray. They may even attempt to negotiate with God, offering to mend their ways in exchange for relief. Severe chronic pain can cause even the most rational among us to try almost anything in the hope of relief. Meditation or prayer seems to help some people to better tolerate pain.

It may be comforting to think that your prayers assist in healing, but according to my dictionary, a "credulous belief in the supernatural" is called "superstition." "Credulous" means believing without much evidence to support it. So let's look at the evidence.

INTERCESSORY PRAYER

Even as Americans paused for the National Day of Prayer and Rememberance, the featured article in the September 2001 issue of the *Journal of Reproductive Medicine*, a respected peer-reviewed medical journal, claimed to have found major health benefits from prayer. "Does Prayer Influence the Success of *In Vitro* Fertilization-Embryo Transfer? Report of a Masked, Randomized Trial" was from the Columbia University Medical Center. Columbia is one of the oldest and most prestigious universities in the nation. The article reported that women who underwent an embryo transfer procedure were twice as likely to become pregnant if they were prayed for without their knowledge by a group of total strangers halfway around the world.

This is "intercessory prayer," prayer offered for others, in this case without their knowledge. That type of intercessory prayer occupies a special place in studies of the power of prayer. Because the person prayed for is unaware that it's happening, intercessory prayer is "blind," and therefore free of the placebo effect. So the patients are not fooling themselves, but what about the researchers? As we saw earlier, Richard Feynman said that science is "what we have learned about how not to fool ourselves."

The first scientist to recognize the importance of blind tests of prayer seems to have been Sir Francis Galton, who in 1872 at the age of fifty published his famous "Statistical Inquiries into the Efficacy of Prayer." Always on the lookout for ways to keep from being misled, Galton was at least a century ahead of his time. It's worth a minute to take a look at this remarkable Victorian scientist and explorer.

THE MAN WHO LOVED TO COUNT

"Whenever you can, count" was a favorite axiom of Francis Galton, and count he did. Realizing while still young that good decisions cannot be made without good information, Galton made a practice of counting everything, even measuring the boredom factor of lectures by counting the number of yawns in the audience. Born into a wealthy and influential family in 1822, he studied medicine at his father's wish, but was dismayed by the lack of data on which to judge whether common medical procedures employed in Victorian England, such as purgatives and bleeding, actually helped.

With the permission of his indulgent father, he switched from medicine to the study of mathematics and statistics at Cambridge. It was fortunate for medicine and the world that he did. He would go on to establish the field of medical statistics, which would be an essential part of the revolution that was about to take place in medical science. Recognizing the capacity of humans for self-deception, Galton played a key role in what is arguably the most important advance in the history of medical research: the randomized placebo-controlled, double-blind trial, by means of which we can know what works and what doesn't. "Statistics," Galton wrote much later, "are the only tools that can cut through the thicket that bars the path of those who pursue the Science of Man."

Galton had an adventurous streak, and his father supported his travels to distant lands to see how others lived. Following the death of his father, who left him a sizeable fortune, he launched a dangerous but highly successful expedition to explore the previously uncharted region of southern Africa now known as Namibia. Exhibiting a trait shared by his equally adventurous cousin Charles Darwin, Galton proved to be a keen observer, making detailed maps and recording the characteristics of the natives—all the while counting everything.

Galton's African adventure was followed by a succession of brilliant ideas: He demonstrated that a person's fingerprints remain unchanged over the years, and devised a practical means of classification that made fingerprinting the indispensable tool in human identification that it remains today. He constructed the first weather maps, which led to daily weather forecasting. Influenced by Darwin, he looked beyond the inheritance of physical characteristics to similarities in intelligence and behavior.

His interest in the heritability of intelligence and behavior led him to develop the statistical methods needed to study them. He found, for example, that identical twins are far more likely to develop similar personalities and interests than are fraternal twins. This is perfectly explicable today in terms of modern genetics, since identical twins are genetically indistinguishable, but the idea that behavior can be inherited as well as learned required a huge intellectual leap in Victorian England, and is still debated today. Twin studies would one day become a major area of psychology research, and Galton was, as always, ahead of his time.

Sometimes he was too far ahead. Galton's reputation today is tarnished, somewhat unfairly, by eugenics, a term he coined for a program to limit reproduction among those characterized as "feebleminded." At the time, however, there was no generally accepted measure of intelligence; the 1916 Stanford-Binet Intelligence Quotient (IQ) was still decades away. Eugenics was widely practiced in the United States in the early twentieth century, and laws calling for sterilization of the mentally deficient were passed in many states. Unfortunately, the laws were often enforced by people who imagined themselves, with little justification, to be at the other extreme of intelligence. It does not help in today's politically correct society that the man who invented eugenics was himself from a relatively privileged segment of society.

The Supreme Court found eugenics laws to be constitutional, but although eugenics laws remain on the books in a number of states, they go unused today. What doomed the eugenics movement was its perversion in Hitler's Germany, where it was used to justify the concept of a master race. Galton devoted the last decade of his life to the eugenics movement, but he was not around to see how it could be distorted in the service of evil. Eugenics is unlikely ever to return, but someday society will have to deal with defective genes.

Galton wrote his famous paper "Statistical Inquiries into the Efficacy of Prayer" in 1872 in response to a published challenge for scientists to devise an experimental test of the power of prayer. Galton, as you might expect, had already done the counting. To satisfy his own curiosity, he had calculated the average longevity of British monarchs and archbishops of the Church of England. Since the Daily Order for Prayer of the Anglican Church calls for prayers for the long life of the monarch and for the archbishop, Galton pointed out that they must surely be the most prayed-for people in all of England.

Because these powerful people would have access to the best medical care, you might expect monarchs and archbishops to live longer than ordinary folk, with or without intercessory prayers on their behalf. Galton, however, discovered that on average they lived no longer than their subjects. Perhaps that reflects the pitiful state of medical knowledge in Victorian England. In any case, as Galton showed, intercessory prayer did not prolong the lives of British monarchs and archbishops.

But the world, particularly the United States, was about to undergo a revival of religious fervor. For more than a hundred years, no other scientist would openly question the power of prayer.

SHARPSHOOTERS AND CHERRY PICKERS

In 1982 Randolph Byrd, MD, a San Francisco cardiologist, enlisted 393 cardiac patients in the San Francisco General Hospital into a double-blind, randomized study to determine whether intercessory prayer, directed to the Judeo-Christian God, had any effect on their medical condition. The patients were randomly assigned to either an intercessory prayer group or to a control group that received no special prayers. Neither patients nor staff knew which group they were in.

The volunteers that did the praying were all born-again Christians, active in local churches. Several were assigned to each patient. They were asked to pray daily for the rapid recovery of the patient and for freedom from complications, including death. No attempt was made to control for additional intercessory prayers offered by family or friends. The results were evaluated in 26 categories, including bacterial infections, congestive heart failure, pneumonia, and the need for diuretics.

In a 1988 paper describing his results, Byrd identified six categories in which the prayed-for group did marginally better. The press reported these six categories as proof of the power of prayer, but of course that leaves twenty categories in which patients did not do better and may have done worse. Statisticians call citing just the data that supports your hypothesis "cherry picking." Scientifically, cherry picking is a sin.

Encouraged by the supposedly positive Byrd study and the media attention it attracted, several other groups undertook prayer studies. They tended to be small studies, with little statistical power and flawed analysis similar to Byrd's cherry picking. Almost all claimed a positive benefit associated with intercessory prayer. The exception was a relatively large study at the prestigious Mayo Clinic involving 799 coronary-care-unit patients. In that statistically powerful study, prayer did not have a significant effect on medical outcomes.

In 1995, with a $600,000 grant from NIH, psychiatrist Elizabeth Targ enrolled 20 patients with advanced AIDS at the University of California, San Francisco Medical Center in a randomized, double-blind pilot study of "distance healing" by the prayers of total strangers. Those selected to pray for the AIDS victims were described as "experienced healers" drawn from a variety of religious traditions.

The study was initiated at a time when AIDS was a death sentence, and the goal was to compare survival times of those who were prayed for with those in the control group. It was expected that most of the advanced AIDS patients would be dead in a few months. Just one month into the six-month trial, however, a new combination of anti-retroviral drugs became standard treatment for AIDS. By the end of the trial, only 1 of the 20 had died. Good news for AIDS victims—bad news for the study.

With the study period now officially over, and the study protocol rendered meaningless, Targ's research team sought to salvage something from the study. They scoured the records of the patients for anything that might indicate that those who had been prayed for fared better. In one category after another, the control group did as well or better than those who were prayed for. Finally, the twenty-third category they examined, "hospital stays and doctor visits," gave a small but statistically significant edge to the prayed-for group. That was the result Targ published. That it was not part of the protocol of the study was never mentioned.

This is a particularly egregious example of what statisticians call the "Texas sharpshooter fallacy." The sharpshooter fires his six-gun at the side of a barn—and then walks over and draws a bull's-eye around the bullet hole.

THE ESP GAP

Targ was a name well known to debunkers of voodoo science. In 1972 at the Stanford Research Institute, physicists Russell Targ and Harold Puthoff announced that they had personally witnessed Israeli psychic Uri Geller using his mind to alter the atomic structure of a metal teaspoon; under nothing but the force of gravity, the mind-altered spoon drooped downward. As James Randi (the Amazing Randi), a stage magician turned fraud buster, has demonstrated countless times since, it is a rather trivial bit of slight-of-hand. With a few minutes of instruction from Randi, even I learned to bend spoons well enough to fool most people. Because of the association of Targ and Puthoff with the prestigious Stanford Research Institute, however, many gullible reporters took the spoon bending confirmation quite seriously, and Geller became an international celebrity.

Scientists who knew Russell Targ scoffed; Targ's eyesight is so notoriously poor, they said, that he would be the last person they would trust to spot any slight-of-hand used by Geller. But although Targ had trouble seeing his hand in front of his face, he was convinced that he could send his mind to view distant places. Puthoff even claimed to have sent his mind to explore the planet Mercury. Who could show he hadn't? Puthoff and Targ wrote about "remote viewing" in their book, *Mind Reach*, and a *Washington Post* columnist invented an "ESP gap" with the Soviets. Scientifically-challenged intelligence officials at the CIA set up a remote-viewing program to exploit the supposed psychic abilities of Targ and Puthoff. So impressed was the CIA by the results that Puthoff and Targ were allowed to recruit additional psychics. The CIA eventually poured hundreds of millions of dollars into efforts to close the ESP gap.

I have never exhibited any natural psychic abilities, but it did enter my mind that there might be a connection between the psychiatrist Elizabeth Targ and the remote-viewing crackpot-physicist Russell Targ. Elizabeth turned out to be Russell's daughter. In his Notes of a Fringe-Watcher column in the *Skeptical Inquirer*, Martin Gardiner noted that Elizabeth's grandfather, William Targ, at one time editor-in-chief at Putnam, also held deep beliefs in the paranormal. Why do people almost invariably adopt the supernatural beliefs of their parents? How much is passed down through the genes? Or is it just that a young brain, soft-wired to learn language, is easily programmed? We'll return to this important question in later chapters.

The story of an intelligent young woman with a PhD who believed that ordinary people could command supernatural forces with just the power of their minds captured the imagination not only of the media, but also of billionaire John Templeton, whom we met in the first chapter. Templeton believes that scientific research should be used to prove the basic tenets of Christianity, and doesn't hesitate to spend his money to make it happen. The John Templeton Foundation had given $5,000 to support Elizabeth Targ's research. Later, in 1997, it supplied $2.4 million to Dr. Herbert Benson to conduct the largest and best-controlled study of intercessory prayer ever undertaken.

Benson was an interesting choice to head the study. We met Benson earlier in this chapter in the discussion of stress reduction. Mind-body medicine tends to be on the outer fringe of modern medicine, but the modest claim of Benson's Mind-Body Medical Institute is: *To the extent that one's medical condition and/or symptoms are caused or made worse by stress, we can help*. Fair enough.

The Benson study included 1,800 heart-bypass patients at six hospitals who volunteered for the study. They were monitored according to strict medical guidelines and randomly assigned either to the group that would be prayed for by anonymous volunteers or to the group that would not. It was a relatively simple protocol that left little room for the sort of manipulation that cast doubt on the results of so many earlier studies on prayer. It was widely predicted that the Benson study would make or break the practice of intercessory prayer therapy. The study was expected to take several years.

THE DOCTOR WHO LOVED THE TRUTH

The Benson Study was underway and the nation was still in mourning for the victims of the 9/11 attack when the September 2001 issue of the *Journal of Reproductive Medicine* arrived in the mail. Bruce Flamm, MD, a clinical professor of obstetrics and gynecology at the University of California, Irvine, opened his copy to the featured article, "Does Prayer Influence the Success of *In Vitro* Fertilization-embryo Transfer? Report of a Masked, Randomized Trial." His endocrine system sprang into action. "I read it and almost fell out of my chair," he remembers.

His grandmother, he recalls, prayed every day for seventy-five years with no success. Unwilling to confront the painful reality that God never answered her prayers, she continually assured her grandson that "prayer can change the world." Still a young boy, Bruce prayed fervently. His prayers, alas, like his grandmother's, went unanswered. In school, on the other hand, he discovered that science always seemed to work. Bruce came to love science and to reject prayer as mere superstition.

The Columbia prayer study in the *Journal of Reproductive Medicine* confronted him with the disturbing realization that an influential medical journal in his own field had just published a paper that was almost certainly superstitious nonsense. The study reported that in vitro fertilization procedures were twice as likely to be successful when the women were prayed for by a group of total strangers halfway around the world. The implication was that such a miracle could be arranged.

News reports of the study, while noting that there were skeptics, treated the finding as genuine science. In its understated style, the *New York Times* called the results "surprising," but if it was true it was more than surprising. It was a miracle.

Arranging miracles, as you can imagine, pays very well. In science, however, there are many surprises but no miracles. Science relies on the principle that there is a physical cause for everything that happens. An ob-gyn with twenty-three years experience in helping women through the amazing process of reproduction, Dr. Flamm was deeply troubled that such a preposterous claim could have passed the peer-review process of a respected journal in his own field. This paper, Flamm suspected, was not merely wrong, but a deliberate fabrication. It was intended only to exploit the religious faith of women who wanted desperately to have a child, with the sole purpose of making money. But how would the authors profit?

To be wrong is not scientific misconduct—few scientists will make it through their careers without making errors. The success and integrity of science rests on a culture of openness, by means of which such errors are eventually exposed and corrected. Scientists have an obligation to call attention to dubious research. As Flamm began digging deeper, he exposed a tangled web of chicanery and deception.

The lead author was Dr. Rugerio Lobo, MD, the chair of the ob-gyn department at Columbia University Medical Center. No one would expect a person in such a position at a distinguished university like Columbia to be involved in deception. Another author, however, Dr. Kwang Cha, a visiting associate professor in the department, was also the wealthy owner of fertility clinics and hospitals in California and Korea, raising serious questions of conflict of interest. But it was the third author that raised Dr. Flamm's blood pressure: Daniel P. Wirth, JD, MS, apparently had no connection to Columbia or to the medical profession. He was a lawyer and a parapsychologist, which is enough to put any scientist on alert. Wirth had a long history of making unsubstantiated faith-based medical claims. What was he doing as a coauthor with certified medical doctors on a "scientific" study at one of the oldest and most respected medical schools in America?

The "Columbia miracle study," as it became known, was widely reported in the public media, including the venerable *New York Times* and *ABC Good Morning America*. A story in the *Times* described the results as showing that faith healing actually works, and copies of the story began showing up in waiting rooms of fertility clinics around the world. It could be seen as an advertisement for the Cha fertility clinics—your clinic might have good doctors, but does it provide proven supernatural help?

The first step should have been for the *Journal of Reproductive Medicine* to immediately withdraw the paper pending an investigation, and for Columbia University to completely disavow the work. Neither happened. Neither the journal nor the university even acknowledged Dr. Flamm's letters relating what he had learned.

Having refused to publish letters critical of the Columbia prayer study, the *Journal of Reproductive Medicine* took the unusual step of publishing a lengthy defense of the study by Dr. Cha. The *Journal* was providing Cha with a platform to defend his study against charges that the *Journal* had adamantly refused even to acknowledge. In his letter, Cha explains that he didn't design the bewildering procedure used in the study—it was Daniel Wirth, the parapsychologist and lawyer, who actually arranged and conducted the study. Any questions must therefore be directed to Wirth.

Daniel Wirth, however, was not available. He had pleaded guilty to unrelated felony fraud charges described in a 46-page federal indictment that extended over a twenty year period, and was on his way to federal prison to serve a 5 year term followed by 3 years of supervised release. How a distinguished institution like Columbia University had become involved with these people remains a mystery.

EXTRAORDINARY CLAIMS

The *Journal of Reproductive Medicine* is a peer-reviewed medical journal. That means papers must be reviewed by anonymous experts before they can be accepted for publication. The identities of the reviewers are closely guarded and they are not compensated for their time; peer review is considered to be a sacred responsibility of scientists. In addition to looking for obvious mistakes, reviewers render their opinion on whether the work is original, whether appropriate credit has been given to previous work, and whether the results are significant enough to warrant publication. The reviewers are expected to treat the material as confidential, and make no personal use of the information until it is in print.

Because a research paper has been peer reviewed does not mean it is right. Reviewers have no way of knowing whether the scientific instruments were functioning properly or if the researchers faithfully reported the results. Clearly, that leaves open the possibility that a peer-reviewed paper contains deliberate fabrication. Although deception does occur, it is extremely rare since every scientific finding must be independently confirmed before it is accepted as new knowledge. Lest we be deceived by faulty tests, scientists must do their testing openly, sharing their findings with other scientists, who are then free to independently replicate every experiment and verify every claim. If the work is fraudulent, eventual exposure is almost certain.

Because science is both open and conditional, errors are self-correcting. Differences between scientists can only be resolved by better experiments—nature is the sole arbiter. In a world addicted to war, no wars are fought over scientific disputes.

"Extraordinary claims," as Carl Sagan put it, "require extraordinary evidence." With the nation still in shock from the 9/11 terrorist attack on the World Trade Center, the Columbia prayer study was treated by many in the media as good news, evidence that God is still in control. In that climate, had the reviewers been unduly deferential to religion? Most scientists were shocked that a reputable journal had chosen to publish it. By what physical mechanism, scientists asked, could a distant prayer influence the penetration of an egg membrane by a spermatozoon? It was certainly an extraordinary claim, but the evidence was anything but extraordinary.

"But couldn't prayer act through some force of which scientists are as yet unaware," a reporter asked me? "There are many things science does not yet know," I replied, "but if someone on their knees somewhere in the world can override natural law by uttering a prayer, there could be no science."

On the day the *New York Times* reported on the Columbia prayer study, I made sure to meet Shaun McCarty and David O'Conner, the two Catholic priests, on their daily walk. I thought David and Shaun would find an experiment to test God offensive. Although always respectful of science, they saw nothing wrong with conducting such experiments, but they were surprised by the result. "God's ways are not our ways," Shaun said. "We cannot always see his purpose." Both Shaun and David had retreated to this line before. Put in other words, I think it means that reality is not always consistent with a wise and loving God.

Meanwhile, on the other side of the continent Dr. Bruce Flamm in California took a darker view of the study. The study actually took place in South Korea. It involved 200 women in Seoul with severe infertility who underwent in vitro fertilization (IVF) in one of Cha's clinics. IVF is the most advanced form of infertility treatment currently available. Half of the women, randomly chosen, were prayed for by Christian volunteers in the United States, Canada, and Australia. The other half received the same IVF procedure, but not the prayers. The praying was done over pictures of the patients that had been faxed to the prayer groups. God would presumably be able to figure out who was being prayed for.

The women being prayed for were separated according to which group, or combination of groups, was doing the praying.

In an effort to amplify the effect, there was a second group praying that the prayers of the first group would be heard. Why not a third group to pray for the second? It all seemed incredibly complicated. Convoluted protocols in statistical studies, such as those used in the Columbia prayer study, are a warning sign. Dividing the entire cohort into smaller subgroups, as they did, increased the odds that a positive effect will be found in at least one subgroup just due to statistical uncertainty. To avoid the cherry-picking fallacy, the number of subgroups must be limited, and to avoid the Texas sharpshooter fallacy, subgroups must be decided on before the study.

Does the God of the entire universe keep score on the number of prayers to decide which are worth answering? You might think a wise and loving God would have some criteria for deciding who should be granted pregnancy other than the size of their support group. But the fact is that no one has a clue as to how God makes his decisions. "God ways are not our ways," as Shaun put it.

Dr. Flamm had other questions. Daniel Wirth was neither a scientist nor a physician. His affiliation was given as a law office. Flamm wrote several letters to the *Journal of Reproductive Medicine* raising questions about the study and about Mr. Wirth's involvement. The responses from the journal were evasive. When Flamm persisted, the journal stopped answering his letters.

Flamm was unrelenting. He published articles in other scientific journals laying out the facts, contacted reporters, protested to influential Columbia alumni, and enlisted scientific colleagues in a letter-writing campaign. After three years of his persistent efforts, the cover-up began to disintegrate.

CRIME AND PUNISHMENT

People outside the scientific community, having heard about the Columbia scandal and Dr. Flamm, began contacting him with more information about Daniel Wirth. Wirth had earlier published several articles about supernatural healing in parapsychology journals. Parapsychology is not regarded as credible by scientists. In 2004, three years after publication of the Columbia prayer study, during which their trial was delayed six times, Wirth and his partner, Joseph Horvath, pleaded guilty in federal court to conspiracy to commit mail and bank fraud involving more than $1 million. Wirth and Horvath were sentenced to five years in federal prison, where Horvath committed suicide. It now appears that Wirth was the organizing force behind the Columbia prayer study.

The lead author, Rogerio Lobo, chair of the ob-gyn department at Columbia, withdrew his name from the paper and later resigned his position. During an investigation by the U.S. Department of Health and Human Services, Columbia University acknowledged that, although he was the lead author on the paper, Dr. Lobo did not even learn of the existence of the study until almost a year after it was completed. It was widely assumed that Dr. Lobo had been forced to step down as department chair because of the scandal surrounding the prayer study. However, he was reassigned to be Director of the Fellowship Program of the Columbia Womens Reproductive Center. Perhaps it was a promotion.

The third author, Dr. Kwang Cha, left Columbia, returning to the management of his fertility clinics in California and Seoul. In February of 2007, Cha was charged by the editor of another journal, *Fertility and Sterility*, with plagiarizing the work of a Korean student in a different paper.

The infamous Columbia prayer study, meanwhile, could still be found on the Web site of the *Journal of Reproductive Medicine*. Indeed, it was still heralded as proof of the power of prayer by fundamentalist Christian publications as far away as Australia. But the worst was yet to come.

On the sixth anniversary of the publication of the study, Dr. Flamm was served with a summons. Dr. Kwang Cha was suing him for "malicious defamation." Cha calculated that Flamm's relentless campaign had cost him millions and demanded a jury trial, no doubt believing a Southern California jury would see Flamm's persistence as the attack of a godless scientist on prayer. The suit threatened to wipe out the retirement fund the Flamms' had slowly accumulated. Even the legal costs involved in defending against such a suit would stretch their resources to the limit. Janice Flamm, already terrified that Daniel Wirth might come after them when he got out of prison, by now only a year away, cried herself to sleep that night.

As this book goes into production, the Flamms are still living under the shadow of Dr. Kwang Cha's defamation lawsuit. Of course, the lawsuit is not about defamation at all. It's an effort to silence criticism of the fraudulent prayer study published in the *Journal of Reproductive Medicine,* a publication coauthored by a notorious con man, currently in federal prison, and a Columbia University professor who now says he had nothing to do with the study. Cha lost the first round. But appealed the decision. It now appears that the lawsuit will go to jury trial. Whatever the final outcome, Dr. Bruce Flamm and his family will have paid a heavy price for his decision as a concerned citizen to expose a fraudulent study masquerading as science.

I asked him if he would do it again. There was a long pause. "I would have to do it," he said softly.

As I write this, the world population clock reads 6,630, 725,709. Most people pray for their health and the health of loved ones. More than a billion pray five times a day. It's a wonder people still get sick.

We are left with the question we began with: can prayer heal?

THE MISSING METRIC

On March 30, 2006, Benson convened a press conference to announce the long-awaited publication in the *American Heart Journal* of the Study of the Therapeutic Effects of Intercessory Prayer. This was the largest and most rigorous study of the efficacy of prayer that had ever been attempted, and it had taken almost a decade. The conclusion of the study was that prayers offered by strangers had no effect on the recovery of people undergoing heart surgery. It will probably be the last major study of the power of intercessory prayer.

The only surprise was that a slight increase in complications was found in a subset of patients who were told that strangers were praying for them. The knowledge that they were being prayed for seemed to interfere with healing. This small, but statistically significant, increase in negative outcomes was attributed by the authors to "performance anxiety." Presumably, being on God's team put them under greater stress. It raised a question about whether it was a good idea to let people know they were being prayed for. Otherwise, there was no difference in the recovery of those who were prayed for and those who were not.

So has science shown that prayer has no effect? Not quite, but the Benson study certainly offers no comfort to those who promote prayer as a solution to the world's problems. Like all studies of prayer, however, the Benson study was of little scientific significance. It was dressed up to look like science, with sigma values attached to probabilities, and control groups, and pages of numbers. As science, however, the Benson study had one unavoidable but fatal flaw. *Prayer has no "metric."*

That's science shorthand for "it can't be measured." We can make some sort of measure of output, for example, a medical evaluation of the patient, but we have no idea how to measure prayer. The *Oxford English Dictionary* defines prayer as "a supplication to a deity," but does it matter which deity? Does it matter whether it is delivered on your knees? Does a prayer for a horse at the racetrack get the same divine attention as a prayer for world peace? Do the prayers of Billy Graham carry more weight than those of a vagrant? Many people no doubt stand ready to offer opinions on these questions, but what evidence could they possibly offer?

CHAPTER FOUR

GIVING UP THE GHOST

In which we search for the soul

Her job description called for her to be a "champion for women's health," and for the five years Dr. Susan Wood served as the head of the Office of Women's Health at the Food and Drug Administration, she was a true champion. In 2005, however, Dr. Wood felt compelled to resign to protest FDA Commissioner Lester Crawford's decision not to approve the emergency contraceptive "Plan B," for over-the-counter sales. The FDA's own scientific advisory panel had overwhelmingly recommended approval.

Since becoming available in the early 1960s, oral contraceptives, fondly called "the pill," have opened doors that had remained shut to women for all of history. Perhaps more than any other single factor, the pill has made it possible for women to be in control of their own lives and to achieve their potential. Today, 100 million women worldwide use the pill. Nevertheless, there are emergencies resulting from rape or failure of contraceptive devices. There are also emergencies resulting from unplanned consensual sex. After all, the human sexual urge was shaped by evolution to ensure procreation, and it works extraordinarily well. Given the right psychological triggers, just about everyone, including presidents of the United States and prominent religious leaders, will risk it all for a forbidden sexual encounter. To insist that society rely solely on abstinence rather than contraception is to deny an instinct against which the gods themselves cannot contend. The entire history of humankind can be read as a testament to the power of that instinct.

Plan B was developed to cover emergencies, whatever their cause. It became available by prescription in 1999. Millions of women have since found Plan B to be safe and effective if taken after intercourse but before a spermatozoon penetrates the membrane of an ovum. This means Plan B must be taken within 72 hours after intercourse. Obtaining a prescription on short notice, however, can be difficult or even impossible, particularly on weekends, which tend to be the most sexually active periods. To avoid delays, and because it is so safe, an FDA advisory panel of medical scientists recommended by a vote of 23–4 that Plan B be made available without prescription.

While the FDA sometimes rejects the recommendations of its expert panels, it had never before done so when a panel vote was so lopsided. Moreover, the FDA's own science staff strongly favored approval. However, one member of the expert panel, Dr. David Hager, a gynecologist from Lexington, Kentucky, with no credentials in medical science, submitted a minority report—a minority of one—in which he equated a fertilized egg with a person.

A leading conservative Christian voice on women's health and sexuality, Hagar's strong opposition to premarital sex and abortion had attracted the attention of the White House, which intervened to have Dr. Hager added to the expert panel. An evangelical Christian, Dr. Hager may have thought it was God who appointed him to the panel. Commissioner Crawford, also an evangelical Christian appointed by Bush, cited Hager's "minority report" as justification for overriding the panel's recommendation. That's when Dr. Wood resigned her post with the FDA.

THE SPARK OF LIFE

I brought up the Plan B controversy with David and Shaun on our next walk. Although we held very different views on family planning, they never seemed in the least offended by my questions. Perhaps they hoped to convert me, or more likely they simply enjoyed, as I did, talking to someone with a totally different worldview, but who shared a desire for a kinder, happier world.

"Why should a fertilized egg be considered a person," I asked? They answered almost in unison: "Because it has a soul." In the eyes of God, they explained to me, this single cell, too small to be seen with the unaided eye, is a human being because God has anointed it. "The miracle of conception compels belief in God," Shaun said a little defensively. "The bestowing of a soul is the spark of life that animates the body and makes it a person. The soul is created at the moment of conception, it defines the person and it survives the person's death."

"Conception is a remarkable event," I conceded. But to myself I was thinking how strange the phrase "spark of life" sounds to a scientist in the twenty-first century. At the beginning of the twentieth century, the existence of a "vital life force" or "divine spark" still seemed necessary to some scientists to explain why some things are mineral while other things composed of the same elements can be alive. This is the ancient concept of vitalism, which long ago lost any meaning in science. The chemistry and physics that animates matter has ceased to be a mystery. Certainly since Watson and Crick resolved the mystery of DNA, there is no longer a need for a "divine spark."

Creation of a zygote from the male and female gametes is nonetheless awesome. The intricate pas de deux of male and female chromosome strands twisting together to form the double helix of a totally unique DNA molecule has a sensuous beauty that inspires reverence.

"Could DNA be the soul," I asked naively? They seemed startled by the suggestion. David, who taught Church law in the seminary, took pride in the relatively enlightened attitude of the Roman Catholic Church toward the findings of science—at least in modern times. He was clearly intrigued by the suggestion that DNA, a material entity that is the focus of modern biology, might be the soul, which has traditionally been thought of as immaterial. He offered to research the question to see if a connection between DNA and the soul had been considered within the Church. Shaun, on the other hand, a poet who taught English literature in the seminary, was unwilling to even consider the suggestion that the soul of a person might be a mere molecule, not even a molecule as marvelous as DNA. "The soul," Shaun said, "is spiritual; it's not a material thing."

In fact, I had been too hasty. People are much more than their DNA. Our personal identity—our "soul" if you insist—keeps changing throughout life as we modify and add to what we believe about the world around us. This change comes not from our genes, but from our culture. In the *Selfish Gene*, Richard Dawkins labeled the units of cultural transmission "memes." They are analogous to genes. Memes, indeed all memories, are stored as real physical changes in the wiring of our brains. They are add-ons to the DNA blueprint.

But a zygote has nothing to remember. It has no sensory apparatus. It therefore feels nothing, sees nothing, hears nothing, and has no brain to store memories if it had anything to remember. The zygote's only function is to divide by mitosis—another awesome process. The result of mitosis is that after perhaps two hours, there will be two cells with identical DNA. In about forty weeks, if all goes well, mitosis repeated over and over will have resulted in a living, breathing human composed of trillions of cells, each one carrying its own copy of the blueprint of the finished person. That, however, is far, far down the road—and all may not go well. No matter how well a marine architect designs a new ship, you can't go to sea in the blueprint. The ship must be built first. It takes more than a unique strand of DNA to make a person.

STEM CELLS

As with the zygote, the only function of the daughter cells resulting from mitosis is to divide again. As the cells multiply, they form a hollow ball called the blastula. The cells of the blastula are undifferentiated. They are not programmed to be muscles, or bones, or anything else. Their only job is to turn out copies. After a few weeks, however, some of the copies begin to exhibit differentiation. They are the first specialists, destined to be part of an eye, or a limb, or an organ. But it is the undifferentiated cells in the blastula that hold the greatest promise for humanity. Scientists are learning how to nudge these undifferentiated embryonic stem cells into becoming whatever specialized cells are needed to overcome various diseases. Initial results show incredible promise for treating or even curing diseases that have tormented humans for all of history.

Moreover, there is an abundant supply of embryonic stem cells. This treasure trove is an unanticipated by-product of the *in vitro* fertilization (IVF) procedure, developed in 1978 by two doctors in the United Kingdom, Patrick Steptoe and Robert Edwards, to treat infertility. Egg cells removed from a woman's ovaries are fertilized outside the body by mixing them with sperm in a liquid medium. A fertilized egg is then transferred to the woman's uterus, where it develops normally. Although religious fundamentalists oppose the IVF procedure as "unnatural," it overcomes most of the obstacles to fertility and has become enormously popular. In the industrialized world, IVF is estimated to account for 1% of all pregnancies.

Normally, the IVF procedure produces far more embryos than are needed. Unused embryos are stored cryogenically in case they might be used for a subsequent pregnancy, or donated to sterile women. An estimated 500 thousand frozen embryos are currently stored in the United States. Perhaps 6 million have been produced. When it becomes clear that frozen embryos will not be needed, they are simply thrown out.

A 1996 law, passed at the urging of right-to-life activists who regard zygotes as people at a very early stage of life, prohibited the use of undifferentiated embryonic stem cells in federally funded research. At the time, the promise of stem-cell research was not widely appreciated by the public, but the law was a serious obstacle to American stem-cell researchers. Harold Varmus, the highly respected director of NIH at that time and a Noble Prize-winning scientist, ruled that the law did not apply to research on stem cells cultured from embryonic tissue in private laboratories. The Varmus rule kept stem-cell research alive in the United States, but it did not please the Bush White House, and Varmus left NIH for the private sector.

As the policies of the Bush administration strayed ever farther from scientific reality, a group of sixty leading scientists, including twenty Nobel laureates, issued a statement charging the administration with manipulating the scientific advisory process. Advisory committees, they charged, were stacked and if they couldn't be stacked, they were disbanded. Advisory committee reports that didn't support the administration position were suppressed, and questionable decisions of federal agencies were shielded from scientific review. The immediate response of the White House to these charges was to trivialize the issue. The elite of the American scientific establishment were dismissed by John Marburger, the top White House scientist, as "a few people with ruffled feathers."

A week later the White House issued a more eloquent response: two advocates of stem-cell research were abruptly dismissed from the Council on Bioethics. They were replaced with appointees who had scant qualifications other than a solid record of faith-based opposition to stem-cell research. The message was clear: if you don't agree with the President, we'll find someone who does.

By 2006 stem-cell therapy was already saving lives. It was just a glimpse of what the future might hold. The mood in Congress and the nation shifted to support of stem-cell research, which was already being more actively pursued in other countries. Nevertheless, there was still strong opposition by religious conservatives. George W. Bush, who owed his narrow reelection victory to the solid support of the religious right, remained firmly opposed to the use of embryonic stem cells in research.

In Rome, Cardinal Trujillo, president of the Pontifical Council for the Family, appeared to speak for Pope Benedict XVI when he threatened Catholics who engage in stem-cell research with excommunication. Italy's most famous stem-cell scientist, Cesare Galli, who had been the first scientist to clone a horse, captured the mood of scientists around the world: "I don't think scientists involved with embryonic stem cell research would care if they are excommunicated or not."

In spite of a veto threat by the president, Congress passed the Stem Cell Research Enhancement Act of 2006. As he had promised, Mr. Bush exercised his veto power for the first time. "The veto was necessary," the president explained in a televised interview, "to protect the dignity of embryos." Instead of being used in research, with the potential to save human lives, the embryos would continue to be thrown out with the garbage— presumably with their "dignity" intact.

Supporters of stem-cell research in Congress did not have enough votes to override the veto. One of the most promising advances in medical history was being held back because of a religious belief that a single zygote cell is endowed with a soul. But what evidence is there for a soul—in a zygote or at any stage of human development?

IN THE BEGINNING

According to a popular joke, a priest, a minister, and a rabbi were discussing the beginning of life. "Life begins at the moment of conception," the priest said. The minister disagreed. "Life does not begin until the fetus can survive outside the mother's womb." The rabbi shook his head. "Every Jew knows that life begins when the last child leaves home and the dog dies."

In most religions, "life" is defined by the existence of a soul, but there is scant agreement on when that happens. Jews and liberal Christians cite Genesis to support their belief that the soul is granted when a newborn infant draws its first breath:

> And the LORD God formed man of the dust of the ground, and breathed into his nostrils the breath of life; and man became a living soul.
>
> Genesis 2:7

But Adam appears to have begun life as a man, not as an infant. That's what makes the Bible such a rich document. The "greatest story ever told" is told through metaphors. People read into those metaphors whatever they wish.

Conservative Christians usually agree with Roman Catholics that a soul is given to the fertilized egg at conception, while most liberal Christians agree with Jews that the soul appears with the first breath. Between conception and birth, every stage of fetal development has been identified with the granting of a soul by some group: when the zygote first divides; when cell differentiation begins; when the embryo contains blood; when the heart first beats; when a brain stem develops; or when the fetus would be viable outside the womb. Biblical passages cited in support of each of these beginnings are clear only to the believers.

If the Bible is the inerrant, divinely inspired word of God, as many believe, why did God choose to be so imprecise? Even when priests, rabbis, and ministers quote the same line of scripture, they notoriously disagree over what it means. They can't all be right—but they can all be wrong.

WHERE HAS BRIDEY MURPHY GONE?

In 1952 Maury Bernstein, an amateur hypnotist in Pueblo, Colorado, put a subject named Virginia Tighe into a deep trance. To his astonishment Virginia began babbling in an Irish brogue and called herself Bridey Murphy. She said she was an Irish woman living in County Cork in the nineteenth century. In numerous subsequent sessions, Virginia (or Bridey) danced

Irish jigs, sang Irish songs, and related Irish stories of her colorful life in County Cork. Bernstein wrote a best-selling book, *The Search for Bridey Murphy*, based on the transcripts of those sessions. It was later made into a movie.

The book and the movie created a sensation. The public couldn't get enough of Bridey Murphy. The story seemed to support the idea of reincarnation in which the soul survives death, not by going to heaven but by transferring to a new body. Just taking count, it would appear that most of the world's population prefers the concept of reincarnation to heaven. Even among those who are nominally Christian, many are fascinated with reincarnation. Hard as life is, people are more interested in being alive than in communing with God. If there is a "God gene," an instinctive belief in God, as some have suggested, it's no match for the survival instinct.

Reporters scoured County Cork in search of any record of a Bridey Murphy, but came up empty. In all the media coverage, however, there is no record of anyone asking the simple question that should have put an end to this whole silly episode right at the start: where had Virginia Tighe's memories of a previous life been stored?

According to Virginia's hypnotic ramblings, Bridey lived not only in a different country, but also in a different century. The real mystery was where Bridey Murphy's memory resided before it was transferred to the wiring of Virginia's brain—not really a very exciting mystery once you take the magic out.

This is the sort of question that separates science from superstition. Information, including memories, must physically reside somewhere or it ceases to exist: Digitally on a computer hard drive, for example, or in the sequence of bases in a DNA molecule, or as marks on 5,000-year-old clay tablets from Mesopotamia, or as connections between human brain cells. Memories can be moved from one storage medium to another, but they're not just floating around waiting to infect someone's brain.

The mystery was finally solved when journalists for the *Chicago American* found Bridey—not in Ireland and not in the nineteenth century, but in Madison, Wisconsin, in the twentieth century. Bridey Murphy Corkell lived across the street from the house in which Virginia Tighe grew up. Virginia's memories were not from a previous life, but from an Irish neighbor in Virginia's own childhood.

Truth is rarely as appealing as well-told fiction, and thousands chose to continue believing the original Bridey Murphy story, and still do. Perhaps, they argue, the *Chicago American* lied. That's a very real possibility, but perhaps nobody lied. A person in a hypnotic trance is under the control of the hypnotist. They will say whatever they believe the hypnotist wants them to say. And the hypnotist may be leading the subject without realizing it.

Not everyone is subject to hypnosis. By some measures, no more than 10% of the population can be put into a deep hypnotic trance. They are frequently people who report profound religious experiences. Hollywood celebrities in particular seem vulnerable to past-life regression under hypnosis, and to belief in reincarnation—and why not? They find being a celebrity addictive. With the helpful guidance of their therapist, celebrities seem invariably to discover that they were celebrities in their earlier lives as well—Cleopatra perhaps or Alexander the Great, never a cobbler or a stablehand.

A reporter asked me how I could be so sure past-life regression is nonsense. "Because there is no verifiable evidence to support it," I replied. That was certainly a true statement, but his response was to shrug his shoulders. "Maybe there is evidence you aren't aware of. Science doesn't know everything." Well, that's true too. I should have said there is no *possibility* of there being valid evidence to support it. There cannot be a gap in the memory chain.

We tend to worry about forgetting things, but vivid memories of things that never happened should also be a concern, and we all have a few such memories. Anecdotal evidence is simply not to be trusted, even when the anecdotes are our own. We must still test and verify.

HARD TIMES IN THE WOMB

Few of us have any recall of events before age three, much less before we were born. And yet it's clear that the very young are acquiring memories at a prodigious rate: memorizing faces, discovering how to get attention, and picking up the first rudiments of language. Everything is new and it's all going into the brain, making wiring connections that may last a lifetime. These early memories might offer insights into our behavior later in life—if they could be accessed.

You will not be surprised to learn that hypnotic regression was employed by therapists to look for early childhood origins of neuroses. Of course they were successful. Soon adults, with the help of their therapists, were recalling the pain of teething and the frustration of being weaned from their mother's breast. But why stop there? Guided by ever-helpful "recovered-memory therapists," people began to recall the warmth and security they had felt in the womb. To the antiabortionists, memories from the womb were all the proof that was needed to make the case that the fetus is a person, complete with feelings and emotions.

Recovered womb memories went over the top in the fall of 1992 when the *San Diego Union-Tribune* published the shocking story of a woman who recalled frightening and painful memories of her mother's unsuccessful attempt to abort her. There is no way to verify that her memories were from the womb, or that they were memories at all. If there is no way to confirm or disprove a claim, there is no reason to attach any significance to it.

GIVING UP THE GHOST

Two hundred years ago there were numerous reports of diaphanous figures rising up from the bodies of persons at the precise moment of their death and ascending toward heaven.

Souls stopped doing that a long time ago, but a hundred years ago Dr. Duncan MacDougall of Haverhill, Massachusetts, constructed an ingenious bed in his office, mounted on a balance platform. It would allow a change in the patient's weight as small as a tenth of an ounce to be detected. A patient near the point of death was placed on the bed and Dr. MacDougall recorded a drop of 21 grams at the moment the man expired, which he attributed to the soul leaving the body. Experiments with several more dying patients produced similar results. Dr. MacDougall acknowledged that his experiment would have to be repeated many times by others to be confident of the result.

He later repeated the measurements several times with dogs, which were apparently poisoned rather than waiting for the inevitable. In the case of dogs MacDougall found no sudden weight loss at death, a finding that confirmed his religious conviction that only humans have a soul. Misguided research has a way of agreeing with the researcher's preconceptions.

MacDougall was also planning to photograph the soul departing the body using an X-ray camera. He reasoned that because an X-ray photograph is a shadow picture, it should image the soul. But before he could get the picture, it was Dr. Duncan MacDougall himself who gave up the ghost.

Although MacDougall's experiments are not regarded today as having any scientific merit and have never been repeated, the figure 21 grams still retains a place in popular folklore as the weight of a human soul. A 2003 film drama nominated for an Academy Award, *21 Grams*, drew its title from the MacDougall result. The search for the soul, however, has moved from avoirdupois to "astral projection."

ASTRAL PROJECTION

Out-of-body experiences have been reported for thousands of years, and there is no reason to doubt that they are real, or at least seem real to the person affected. They are often associated with hallucinogenic drugs or neurological conditions such as migraine headaches and epilepsy. Such an episode typically involves a strong impression of being apart from your body, often floating above it. This is particularly powerful if it occurs as part of a near-death experience. To the religious, who believe in the existence of a soul that survives the body, it is easy to imagine that their soul has departed their dying body and is hovering above the deathbed, looking down.

To New Age believers, reports of out-of-body experiences confirm their conviction that consciousness is something apart from the body that can gather information from distant places, as in remote viewing, and return with it to the body. They refer to this as "astral projection." The tabloid media has a particular fascination with out-of-body experiences, and even the CIA bought into it during the height of the Cold War, spending millions of dollars to put together a group of remote-viewing psychics at CIA headquarters in Langley, Virginia. They claimed to be able to project their minds anywhere. Reportedly, they were able to project themselves into the Kremlin, but could never get quite close enough to read documents. That the CIA is so easily conned is scary.

To scientists, none of this makes any sense. They're inclined to see out-of-body experiences as just another misperception of a brain that must reconcile a number of sensory inputs. In particular, scientists automatically reject any mystical interpretation such as the soul. Their conviction is that when we better understand how the brain processes sensory information, out-of-body experiences will no longer seem strange.

In fact, that's already happening. In 2006, two patients, both women, were being evaluated for epilepsy surgery at University Hospital in Geneva. Doctors implanted dozens of electrodes in their brains to pinpoint the abnormal tissue that was causing their seizures. Dr. Olaf Blanke, a Swiss neurologist, reported in the journal *Nature* that mild electrical stimulation of a region in the brain called the angular gyrus induced out-of-body experiences in both patients. Both women, who had normal psychiatric histories, found the experience disturbing and unpleasant. One felt she was hanging from the ceiling; the other felt there was a shadowy person behind her interfering with her actions.

Located in the parietal lobe, the angular gyrus is in a multisensory region of the brain involved in a number of processes related to cognition. It processes information from the primary senses to tell the brain where the body is positioned in space. There are far more senses involved than the five we learn about in school. We have balance organs in our ears to keep us upright, and millions of sensors in our skin are constantly mapping heat and cold over the entire body. Nerves in our joints and tendons relay stresses to the brain. The brain must make sense of this jumble of signals, but the brain can easily be duped.

A year after the brain stimulation experiments, Dr. Blanke found that the out-of-body experiences could be induced without brain stimulation or hallucinogenic drugs. The subject was fitted with display goggles that showed a video image of the person from a different perspective. The subject's brain would buy into the illusion very quickly.

The work of Dr. Blanke and others had no impact on the paranormal community, which continues to cite out-of-body experiences as proof that consciousness exists apart from the body.

The soul, or spirit, plays an important role in virtually every religion on earth. But the spirit divides rather than unites. Disputes over the soul remain unresolved because there are no facts, only unsupported beliefs. There is, however, one place we have not yet looked—heaven. If we can find evidence of heaven, there must be souls to fill it. In the next chapter we will look for heaven.

CHAPTER FIVE

THE SILENT ARMY

In which we search for an afterlife

The grey figures of the life-size terra-cotta warriors seem to swallow up the artificial light beneath the huge dome that covers the excavation. They stand there in the gloom, column after column in battle formation, weapons in hand. Seeing them for the first time, you find yourself speaking in the hushed tones people use at funerals, but the funeral was 2,200 years ago. The army was assembled to guard the first emperor of all China in the afterlife.

The Chinese have a tragic history of granting too much power to their leaders, and Qin Shi Huang's power was absolute. The secret of maintaining absolute power is to keep the people ignorant of the outside world. People will accept total servitude only as long as they believe it is the normal condition. The Great Wall of China, completed by Qin, is symbolic of the obsession with isolation in imperial China.

In today's world, however, walls that cannot be breached by armies are easily penetrated by radio waves. Isolation in the modern world requires control of the media, which is called on in dictatorships to spew out incessant propaganda. In 1966, the revolutionary hero Mao Zedong, who had lost much of his influence as a result of the failure of his hopelessly impractical Great Leap Forward, launched the terrifying Great Proletarian

Cultural Revolution in a desperate effort to regain power. He recruited a militia of young Chinese zealots called the Red Guard, imbued them with patriotic fervor, and unleashed them on his political foes.

THE MANDATE OF HEAVEN

In the history of governance, the inheritance of authority by the offspring of the sovereign must surely be both the most widely practiced and least rational method of choosing a leader. Its only virtue was to minimize squabbling over succession, but even that frequently had rather notorious failures. Not surprisingly, kings and emperors invariably discovered that their legitimacy had actually been conferred by a higher power. The European notion of the divine right of kings is spelled out rather nicely in the New Testament:

> *Let every soul be subject unto the higher powers. For there is no power but of God: the powers that be are ordained of God. Whosoever therefore resisteth the power resisteth the ordinance of God: and they that resist shall receive to themselves damnation. For rulers are not a terror to good works, but to the evil. . . . But if thou do that which is evil, be afraid: for he beareth not the sword in vain: for he is the minister of God, a revenger to execute wrath upon him that doeth evil.*
>
> Romans 13:1–4

However the king is chosen, and even if he turns out to be a homicidal maniac, he's still the one in charge according to this scripture. Kings no doubt loved the part about the "revenger," where the king gets to "execute wrath." The amount of human suffering these verses have sanctioned over the centuries is hard to imagine.

Except in the Muslim world, kings have long since been stripped of any real authority. It's an embarrassment to rational pretensions that many otherwise modern nations still cling to their royal families for ceremonial purposes.

The traditional Chinese concept of sovereign rule, known as the Mandate of Heaven, is similar to the divine right of kings, but it at least adds an escape clause allowing the overthrow of unjust emperors. Heaven would bless the authority of a just ruler, but would be displeased with an unwise ruler and give the mandate to rule to someone else. Paradoxically, while it was considered wrong to revolt, a successful insurrection was accepted as evidence of heaven's approval.

Insurrections were often led by natural leaders of humble birth, who would then become emperor, founding a new dynasty. The new emperor and his immediate offspring might be relatively enlightened. But the corrupting influence of absolute power would, after a few generations, produce increasingly intolerable despots. Their overthrow would mark the start of yet another dynasty.

Although Mao officially declared an end to the Cultural Revolution in 1969, it had by then taken on a life of its own: violence, denunciations, public humiliations, and mass executions continued until 1976, the year Mao died. With Mao, however, hereditary succession in China seems to have come to an end. It now seems inconceivable that it will ever return. Someday, when memories of the terror inflicted by the Red Guard have faded, Mao may be remembered as a hero who brought an end to hereditary rule in China.

All of this happened virtually out of sight. Nearly a fourth of the world's population was isolated behind a bamboo curtain. The historic visit of President Richard Nixon to Beijing in 1973, during which he met with Mao, lifted the corner of the bamboo curtain just enough to give the world its first televised glimpse of The People's Republic of China in seven years. It was a shock. China had become the most exotic country on Earth—and the most backward.

But as the world got a peek at the horror in China, so also the Chinese people got a glimpse of the modern world. They coveted what they saw. Once contact, however tenuous, had been established with the outside world, Mao's final revolution was doomed.

LETTING IN THE LIGHT

After more than two thousand years of total darkness, the emergence of Qin's terra-cotta army into the light just one year after Nixon's visit is a metaphor for China's transformation from the backwardness of the Great Leap Forward and the madness of the Cultural Revolution into a modern industrialized nation.

The greatest archaeological find of the twentieth century, perhaps of all time, the terra-cotta army of Qin Shi Huang was discovered in 1974 by peasants digging a well not far from Qin's tomb. Only a few hundred of the terra-cotta figures had been uncovered when I was taken to the site a few years later as a member of a scientific delegation from the University of Maryland.

Since that time, more than 8,000 life-size terra-cotta warriors and horses, strategically deployed to guard Qin's tomb, have been unearthed. These soldiers are not mass-produced look-alikes, turned out of a mold like a child's toy soldiers. No two are alike. The various battalions even exhibit different racial features, reflecting the widespread regions that had been united under Qin. They were individually sculpted from living soldiers in Qin's vast army. It was remarkably enlightened for the time—Qin could have chosen to have the army buried alive.

Qin Shi Huang was the most powerful man in the world. He could have anything he desired no matter what it cost. Yet much of the wealth of his empire was squandered on the one thing he could not buy: an extension of his power beyond the grave. Quite independently, the pharaohs in Egypt had constructed the Great Pyramids for the same reason.

In China at the time of Qin, religion in the Western sense simply did not exist. There were plenty of oracles, magic healers, and wise elders full of advice on how to avoid offending the spirits, but no word for religion existed in the Chinese language. For the masses there were neither places of worship nor priests to intercede with heaven. The emperor filled the role of God for his subjects, but unlike the all-powerful gods of Western religions, Qin would need an army in the afterlife to maintain the status he had in this life. Emperors and pharaohs had both tasted absolute power. Small wonder they would seek to arrange the same advantages in the next life that they enjoyed in this one.

There have been no reports from the other side to indicate how well they succeeded, and yet belief in an afterlife is almost universal. Americans profess belief in an afterlife in the same sort of overwhelming numbers that claim to believe in the existence of God. Polls, however, do not measure depth of conviction. What would those who profess to believe in Heaven be willing to wager on it?

LITTLE DUCKY DADDLE

In 1997, thirty-nine members of Heaven's Gate, a secretive New-Age UFO cult in San Diego, committed ritual mass suicide in the belief that their souls would be taken on board a huge spaceship that they believed was hiding behind Comet Hale-Bopp. The spaceship, they believed, would take them to the Kingdom of Heaven. We are unable to explain why they held this belief, or why they felt compelled to demonstrate the depth of their conviction. Nevertheless, they passed the test.

Surely there must be some way short of mass suicide by which people can prove their faith. But where is the evidence that leads so many people to declare their belief in heaven? You can fill a library with books on the subject, but they all end up in the same place. To the question, "How do we know heaven exists?" Ralph Muncaster of the Evidence of God Ministries begins:

> First we have to agree on the authority of the Bible. Once we agree on the authority of the Bible, we can examine what the scripture says about heaven.

Well, there you have it. There is a Heaven because the Bible says there is a heaven.

"Jesus loves me this I know, for the Bible tells me so," went the song we sang in Sunday school. It was the first song I ever learned. As most Christian children do, I learned it before I learned to read. It's taught early, before our brains get filled up with conflicting ideas.

I expect you can remember the first two songs you learned, but probably not the third. I learned my second song, "Little Ducky Daddle," when I got to kindergarten:

> A little ducky daddle went wading in a puddle,
> Went wading in a puddle quite small.
> It really doesn't matter, how much I splash and splatter,
> I'm just a ducky daddle after all.

On long drives my father would ask me if I could sing "Ducky Daddle" for him once again. He said it was his favorite song. I would stand behind him on the floorboards of the Model A, holding on to the back of his seat, and sing "Ducky Daddle" over and over. I can still remember the songbook with a picture of the happy little duckling walking in the rain with an umbrella—a little rain doesn't matter. Everything we will learn for the rest of our lives must first be reconciled with these early childhood lessons. Because there are few conflicting ideas at that age, the thalamus routes them directly to the amygdalae. Everything children learn in those early years matters.

Muncaster goes on to explain that heaven is mentioned 580 times in the Bible, "so clearly God wants us to understand its importance." All of a sudden we're no longer talking about whether heaven exists. The question of whether it exists has been replaced by whether the Bible is the authority.

"Science rejects appeal to authority in favor of empirical evidence," federal Judge John E. Jones wrote in his 2005 opinion in *Kitzmiller v. Dover Area School Board*, discussed in chapter 2. That one line goes to the heart of the conflict between science and religion. Science rejects authority, and religion is built on it. This was the key to the conclusion of Judge Jones that intelligent-design theory is not, as it claims to be, a scientific theory.

LOOKING FOR HEAVEN

On the day Judge Jones issued his opinion, I clicked on the television to the *ABC Evening News* to assess the media reaction. Embedded in the news was a promotion for an ABC news special that would be shown later that evening, *Heaven: Where is it? How do we get there?*, a two-hour special with popular interviewer Barbara Walters. More than a year in the making, it was a coincidence that *Heaven* was to be aired just hours after the landmark *Kitzmiller* church-state decision. Something is stirring in the land. Religion in America is going through an uneasy transition. The conflict with rationality has broken out in the open.

How, I wondered, would ABC fill two hours of valuable prime time on a subject about which nothing at all is known? If you're Barbara Walters, it's easy: you interview celebrities, from actor Richard Gere, who says he's a Buddhist, to California's first lady, Maria Shriver. Do they know anything about heaven? Not a thing. Nevertheless, the public wants to hear from celebrities. Throw in a few interviews with religious leaders such as the Dalai Lama, who is also something of a celebrity these days, a couple of scientists to give people a chance to relieve themselves, a few delusional people who imagine they've been there, and you've covered everything that's known about heaven in less time than it takes to watch the Super Bowl. That's because we really don't know anything.

The only hard information in the two hours came in the introduction. An ABC News poll reported that 90% of the public believes in heaven—whatever it is. That tells us a lot about the public, but not much about heaven. Other polls have reported about the same percentage for several years, including a respected Harris poll just a year earlier. Like most opinion polls, however, the numbers give little idea of the depth of conviction. Why isn't there a stampede to buy tickets? In spite of all the pain and disappointment that comes with it, it's this life that people want.

Although almost everyone interviewed agreed that there is an afterlife, there was no agreement on what it's like. Cardinal Theodore McCarrick, archbishop of Washington DC, told Barbara Walters that Catholics believe the body is physically resurrected and we will be reunited with loved ones. A leader of American Muslims was much more specific: silken couches and the delights of fine food, wine, and sex.

The most revealing contrast was between mega-church evangelist Ted Haggard and a failed Muslim suicide bomber in a Jerusalem prison. Haggard was certain that heaven is strictly for born-again Christians, while the would-be suicide bomber was just as certain that heaven is only for Muslims. Just a year after his appearance on the *Heaven* special, Haggard was forced to resign as president of the National Association of Evangelicals when he admitted buying the street drug meth from his male prostitute. Are these among the delights of heaven?

EYEWITNESS ACCOUNTS

I met with David O'Conner and Shaun McCarty the day after the federal court ruling in the Dover case to get their take. We had not gone on our regular walks beside the millstream for almost a year. Complications from a severe case of flu had left David connected to an oxygen tank. I feared he would never be free of it, but on this day he met me at the door without the oxygen mask. He was greatly improved and in good spirits. It was Shaun who did not seem well. His voice, always very soft, was now almost inaudible. I strained to make out what he was saying, but I'm not sure how much of that was my growing deafness since my encounter with the tree.

The conversation, however, quickly turned from evolution to the Barbara Walter news special on heaven. Shaun, who had come close to dying from colon cancer a few years earlier, thought the most convincing part of the program was the interviews with people who have had a near-death experience. It seems that there is nothing like having been there, however briefly, to make you a believer in heaven. A widely quoted 1997 feature article in *U.S. News & World Report* put the number of Americans who have near-death experiences at 15 million. It sometimes seems as if all of them have written a book about it, and many of the accounts seem similar—if you're looking for similarities. They often include being in a long tunnel with a bright light at the end, and feelings of contentment.

Accounts of near-death experiences have been around for thousands of years, but modern resuscitation techniques have made them much more common. For a scientist, however, it's hard to imagine less reliable evidence. It is based solely on memory with no physical evidence. Worse, it is the memory of a time when the person was not only unconscious, but whose brain cells were beginning to die and wildly misfiring. It's like seeking religious insight in the hallucinations induced by peyote. Of course, many people do attach religious significance to peyote-induced hallucinations.

We have a well-documented tendency to confound what we are seeing with what we remember. They are not always the same. When an image is obscured, the brain tends to fill in the picture with images stored in the memory. Having heard stories of the tunnel and the light, people are perhaps more inclined to describe their own near-death hallucinations in a similar way.

Most of the judgments we are forced to make in life are based on insufficient evidence. This can be very uncomfortable. People long for something or somebody to tell them what to do, or what to believe. They find countless ways to avoid the hard work of thinking. Some will turn to Ouija boards, some to horoscopes, and others to peyote. In any case, a glimpse of heaven is not to be found in the feeble flickering of a dying brain.

WHAT DO WE REALLY WANT?

While the Christian Bible may mention heaven 580 times, it offers no hint about what it's like. Only scoundrels and lunatics claim to receive messages from beyond the grave, and of course no such claim has ever been verified. If there is an afterlife, it remains totally hidden from the living.

In the absence of any prospect of experimental verification, the question of an afterlife cannot be the subject of scientific discussion. But in his second encyclical letter to the faithful, "On Christian Hope," Pope Benedict XVI asks a more valid question: "Do we really want this—to live eternally?" The question reveals a totally unexpected side to this pope. As Cardinal Ratzinger, before his election as pope, he headed the Congregation for the Doctrine of the Faith, the Vatican office previously known as The Holy Office of the Inquisition. Thus he was the official defender of traditional Catholic doctrine, even characterizing the Church's persecution of Galileo as "reasonable and just."

However, his second encyclical as pope, issued on November 29, 2007, could have come from the Enlightenment. "The atheism of the nineteenth and twentieth centuries," he wrote, "is—in its origins and aims—a type of moralism: a protest against the injustices of the world and of world history."

On the question of whether we really want eternal life, he wrote:

> Perhaps many people reject the faith today simply because they do not find the prospect of eternal life attractive. What they desire is not eternal life at all, but this present life, for which faith in eternal life seems something of an impediment. To continue living for ever—endlessly— appears more like a curse than a gift. Death, admittedly, one would wish to postpone for as long as possible. But to live always, without end—this, all things considered, can only be monotonous and ultimately unbearable.
>
> . . . To eliminate [death] or to postpone it more or less indefinitely would place the earth and humanity in an impossible situation, and even for the individual would bring no benefit. Obviously there is a contradiction in our attitude, which points to an inner contradiction in our very existence. On the one hand, we do not want to die; above all, those who love us do not want us to die. Yet on the other hand, neither do we want to continue living indefinitely, nor was the earth created with that in view. So what do we really want? Our paradoxical attitude gives rise to a deeper question: what in fact is "life"?

What indeed? Scientists at the J. Craig Venter Institute in Rockville, Maryland, announced that they had "built from scratch" a synthetic chromosome containing all the genetic material needed to produce a primitive bacterium. This puts them tantalizingly close to creating an artificial form of life that can replicate itself. Venter predicted they will succeed within the year. This has been done using only off-the-shelf chemicals. The concept of a divine spark or vital life force now seems meaningless. Life is just chemistry.

CHAPTER SIX

THE TSUNAMI GOD

In which the innocent suffer

In North America it was Christmas day. On the other side of the world in Banda Aceh, Sumatra, it was the morning of December 26, 2004. It was a beautiful day in a beautiful land. Children played on the beach, mothers prepared breakfast, fisherman set out in their boats. When the ground shook, people rushed outside to look and to call their children, but there was no significant damage, and they soon went on with their day. A few people who happened to look westward over the Indian Ocean, however, noticed a strange line stretching along the horizon.

When the ocean is calm and the air is clear, an adult of average height standing at the water's edge sees the horizon about three miles away. But the ocean that day was not as calm as it appeared. As people watched, the water's edge began receding from the beach. A huge wave was headed toward shore at the speed of a jetliner. Waves travel faster in deep water. As water becomes shallower nearer shore, the water at the foot of the wave is slowed down by friction with the ocean bottom, causing the leading edge to become ever steeper. This is why surf breaks on beaches—the tops of the waves outrun the bottoms. No matter what direction waves travel farther out, to a person on the beach it appears that waves always arrive almost perpendicular to the shore. This is the phenomenon of refraction. As the wave approaches the beach at an angle, the part of the wave that is in deeper water moves faster than the part of the wave in shallower water. This causes the wave to change direction, turning toward the shore.

The first wave that struck the beach at Banda Aceh was a gigantic surge, almost a hundred feet high. Waves continued to surge ashore at intervals of about thirty minutes, disrupting any rescue efforts. The third wave was the largest, after which they gradually diminished. But for the rest of the day the waves prevented any organized rescue.

Banda Aceh was the first heavily populated area on the Sumatra coast hit by the tsunami. The scene was repeated along thousands of miles of coastline around the Indian Ocean. There was a death from the tsunami as far away as Port Elizabeth, South Africa, more than five thousand miles from the epicenter. The total of dead and missing from the tsunami would approach three hundred thousand. The victims were disproportionately those of small stature who were less able to withstand the surging water—children.

As the world launched a massive disaster-relief effort, the question people everywhere asked was, what had caused the tsunami?

ACTS OF GOD

Aceh, which was the region hardest hit by the tsunami, is a fundamentalist Islamic society, which in recent years has been torn by armed conflict between Aceh separatists and the Indonesian army. Westerners, particularly European tourists who frequent other parts of Indonesia, stay away from Aceh because of the fighting. As in other fundamentalist Islamic regions of the world, anti-American sentiment was strong, and rumors quickly spread that the tsunami was a test of a new American weapon.

This sort of anti-American conspiracy theory is seemingly inevitable when bad things happen in the Muslim world. Fundamentalist Islamic clerics had to choose between blaming the disaster on America or on the sinful practices of the populace. They chose to emphasize sin, attributing the death and destruction to punishment meted out by Allah to those who neglect the teachings of the Qur'an.

In a television interview posted on the Internet by the Middle East Media Research Institute, a professor at the Al-Imam University in Saudi Arabia explained that Allah permits the collective destruction of villages and cities if sin is rampant: "The fact that it happened at Christmas time, when corrupt people from all over the world gather at beach resorts to commit fornication and sexual perversion, is a sign from Allah."

The word "Islam" means "submission." To many Muslims, enduring pain or loss is a way of submitting to the will of Allah. Perhaps people had shirked their daily prayers, or followed a materialistic lifestyle. Women who had been seen in public without the *hijab*, or head covering, in the period before the disaster were singled out for scorn and paraded through coastal villages. Three hundred thousand dead may seem to be excessive punishment for a few women exposing their hair, but who are we to judge God? Satan and his jinn are allowed to inflict suffering and adversity not only as punishment for moral lapses, but also as a test of humility and faith.

In Western law, any natural calamity, whether a tsunami that kills hundreds of thousands or a tree that falls on a single runner, is classified as an act of God, meaning no one can be held legally responsible for its consequences. However, there is a long tradition among both Christians and Muslims of punishing individuals thought to be responsible for bringing down the wrath of God on a community. We no longer burn witches at the stake for causing disease or crop failure, but as recently as 2006, televangelist Pat Robertson, with a following of millions, was calling on God to unleash hurricanes on sinful Florida. God is certain to oblige his request—it's only a matter of when. Indeed, if being in the path of hurricanes is the measure of sin, Florida has been sinful since they first began keeping weather records. Robertson also suggested that Dover, Pennsylvania, could expect to be hit by natural disasters for voting fundamentalist school-board members out of office.

By this way of thinking, there are no natural disasters. All disasters are supernatural. That would be consistent with both the Bible and the Qur'an, neither of which recognizes the existence of natural laws that operate independently of God's will. All that happens in the world is God's doing. In the eleventh century, the Islamic imam al-Ghazali argued that cause and effect is not allowed since it would limit the freedom of Allah to bring about whatever events he wants. This was accepted as Islamic sacred law and so remains today.

Should we therefore assume that all three hundred thousand victims of the tsunami were being punished for their sins, or does God accept collateral damage in the form of innocent victims as the necessary price of divine retribution? Indeed, the Old Testament God of Abraham never shirked his responsibility to punish sinners just because it would also inflict suffering on the innocent. He does so repeatedly in the Old Testament— and appears to continue to do so today.

Far from the Indian Ocean, a leading Muslim cleric in Southern California saw the tsunami as "a test from God to see how humans respond." The explanation of natural disasters as divine tests to measure worthiness seems to be accepted by all religions. The reward for being blameless presumably lies in the next life. In Edward Fitzgerald's version of the Rubaiyat, the skeptical Omar Khayyam advises, "Ah, take the cash and let the credit go."

As the tsunami reached one shore after another around the Indian Ocean, it was not just Muslims who suffered. The inhabitants of poor fishing communities along the southern coast of India are Hindus. They worship local deities, most of whom are female, as well as the major Hindu gods such as Shiva. These local gods have the power to destroy as well as create.

The ocean itself is seen as a terrible god who eats people and boats, but also provides food. Hindu fishermen seek to calm the angry god by acts of propitiation. Rather than feeling personal guilt, they are more inclined to assume that a natural disaster is punishment for misdeeds they committed in a previous life.

Along the coastline of Thailand and Sri Lanka, also hit hard by the tsunami, the population is overwhelmingly Buddhist. But it's not quite the philosophical Buddhism of contemplation and acceptance that so many educated Westerners are drawn to. While worshiping no single supreme being, ordinary Buddhists have many weather gods they can blame who must be propitiated with prayers and offerings. Only in retrospect do Buddhists reflect on karma and ask what they had done that led to such a tragedy.

There are at least as many people in the world who believe in reincarnation as people who believe in heaven. Asked how we should view a disaster that claimed the lives of perhaps two hundred thousand innocent children, a Buddhist leader in Southern California shrugged that "children are not innocent—you can be punished at any time for misdeeds in a previous life." Reincarnation thus serves as a convenient explanation for the suffering of innocents. Life itself is suffering brought about by attachment to worldly things. Disasters, in the Buddhist view, should be seen not as punishment but as something for people to rise above. In this sense, a natural disaster becomes a test. A good grade on the test generates merit for the next life.

Christians and Jews were a small minority among those directly affected by the tsunami. Unlike the Muslim imam al-Ghazali, Christian and Jewish theologians long since reconciled God and natural law. Medieval rabbi Moses Maimonides reasoned that armed with foreknowledge, God chooses to achieve his purposes using natural law. Because we mere mortals cannot see into the future, we cannot expect to understand why God allows certain things to happen. At about the same time, Saint Thomas Aquinas reached a similar conclusion, arguing that as a matter of faith we must accept that disasters are the reflection God's love for us. There are obvious pitfalls of circular reasoning in this argument, but at least Maimonides and Aquinas make room for natural law and thus for science.

A thousand years, however, seems to be too short a time for this concept to filter down to the masses. From Christian pulpits around the world, the tsunami was compared to God's test of Job. Writing in the *New York Times*, conservative columnist William Safire, a Catholic who has pretensions as a theologian, was among those invoking the biblical account of Job to explain why an all-powerful and loving God had not intervened to prevent the suffering of innocents. It's worth a minute to review this curious tale.

JOB IN TEXAS

Like most of the other children attending Sunday bible class at the Methodist church in Donna, Texas, I was there because it pleased my mother. Sunday school, like natural disasters, is something that must be endured. Under the circumstances, I tried to make the best possible use of the time by daydreaming of distant adventures, only occasionally tuning in on the lesson.

One of the few lessons that interrupted my daydreaming was the story of Job, described by the teacher as one of the most important stories in the Bible. Indeed, Christian and Judaic scholars have been trying to make sense of the Book of Job for a thousand years. As we will see, they haven't gotten very far.

The story is familiar to those from a Judeo-Christian culture. As related by my Sunday-school teacher:

> *There lived in the land Uz at about the time of Moses a good man named Job. Job served the Lord God faithfully, and prayed to him every day. He was the richest man in the land with thousands of sheep, and oxen, and camels. God pointed him out to Satan as "a perfect man who fears God and does nothing evil."*

Not impressed, The Evil One questions the depth of Job's devotion:

"Of course Job praises God; you blessed him and made him a rich man. Take it all away and he will curse thee to thy face." Stung by Satan's words, God accepts the wager, allowing Satan to do with Job's sons and possessions whatever he wishes, forbidding him only from harming Job's person.

Job soon learns that savages from the desert have driven away the work animals and killed the men that were plowing and working with them. No sooner does he learn this than he is told that lightning has killed all his sheep and the shepherds tending them, and enemies from Chaldea have taken away all the camels and killed the men who were with them. Then another messenger arrives with even worse news: Job's sons and daughters had met together to eat and drink in the house of his oldest son when a great wind from the desert collapsed the house, killing them all. In one day Job had lost everything. He threw himself on the ground before the Lord and said: "Naked came I out of my mother's womb, and naked I will return. With nothing I came into the world, and with nothing I shall leave it. The Lord gave and the Lord hath taken away; blessed be the name of the Lord."

God could not refrain from crowing to Satan that he had won the wager:

"Hast thou considered my servant Job? He holds fast to his goodness, even after I let you do him great harm."

Satan, however, easily bamboozles God a second time:

Satan answered the Lord, "All that a man has he will give for his life. Harm his person and he will curse thee to thy face." Again God gives Job over to Satan, this time asking only that Satan spare Job's life.

Satan afflicted Job with sores from the sole of his foot to the top of his head. Job was in great pain, but would not speak one word against God. Even Job's friends believed that he must have done some terrible thing to make God so angry. But still Job remained faithful, and refused to say that God had dealt with him unjustly. Though he did not understand God's ways, Job still believed that God was good.

This remarkable tale of suffering and faith called out for a Hollywood-style ending in which virtue is rewarded and the hero lives happily ever after. The final verse was almost certainly added much later, perhaps by a translator:

God himself then spoke to Job and his friends, telling them that it is not for man to judge God, and that God will do right by every man. And so God makes it right, curing Job of his sores and making him richer than ever with more than twice as many sheep, oxen, and camels as before. And he gave Job seven more sons and three daughters who were said to be the loveliest women in the land. And Job lived a long life in riches, and honor, and goodness under God's care.

So there we have it. The God of Abraham does not come off in the Book of Job as a kindly shepherd tending his flock, but as a vain and boastful god, easily manipulated by the taunting of Satan. This is a god more in the image of the Greek gods, with exaggerated human failings. Or so it seemed to me as a boy when I listened to the story of Job for the first time in Sunday school.

Never once was it suggested that perhaps the Book of Job was an allegory, or that Job was not an actual historical figure. The Sunday-school teacher drew three lessons from the Book of Job: (1) We must not judge God; (2) we must hold to our beliefs in spite of overwhelming evidence to the contrary; and (3) God will reward us for this—but perhaps not in this life.

One girl in the class was moved to tears by the story. "Job hadn't done anything wrong," she wept, "it's just not fair. It wasn't enough that God eventually gave everything back," she said between sobs, "you can't undo pain." Others in the class agreed with her.

I was troubled for a very different reason. Why was it all about Job? What of Job's children, who died in the windstorm, and his servants who were murdered by the savages? Or even his innocent livestock? Their lives were not restored. Had they been sacrificed just to settle a wager?

Theologians will protest at this point that Job is not history. It's an allegory that strives to make sense of the bad things that happened in the world in a time before science. Exactly! But we weren't told that. Most of the population is convinced that the Bible is the inerrant word of God.

So why did the Indian Ocean tsunami happen?

THE TECTONIC PISTON

For scientists, whose business it is to understand why things happen, natural disasters become experiments. While religious leaders pondered questions of divine punishment and whether humans are subjected to testing by some supernatural intelligence, geophysicists were studying the data from seismic stations around the world. A gigantic earthquake centered in the Indian Ocean about a hundred miles west of Sumatra was the proximate cause of the tsunami. But what had caused the earthquake?

It was one of the most powerful earthquakes recorded since the invention of the modern seismometer. We live on the thin, solid crust of a molten planet that has been cooling since it was formed 4.5 billion years ago. The crust is broken up into tectonic plates, great slabs of rock that push against one another along fault lines as Earth continues to cool. Occasionally the plates fracture or slide over one another. Earthquakes are abrupt movements of these tectonic plates along the fault lines.

Like a stick bent until it snaps, elastic energy built up between two major plates in the Indian Ocean was suddenly released as one plate abruptly slid over the other. Not every quake below the ocean results in a major tsunami, but because one tectonic plate was forced upward by the movement, it acted like a giant piston, pushing up a huge volume of water. The water spread out across the ocean in concentric ripples, like pouring a pail of water into a pond.

Tectonic earthquakes are an inevitable natural phenomenon. On a smaller scale, they occur somewhere in the world every day. This one was simply much larger than most. Nevertheless, because it was centered far out at sea, the earthquake itself caused little damage. Although the waves were very high, they were also very wide, so that ships at sea experienced only a gentle rocking as the tsunami passed beneath them. The devastation came when the waves reached the shoreline.

The tragedy was that in the time between the earthquake and the arrival of the tsunami at Banda Aceh, there was plenty of time for people to seek higher ground—if they had known. The shock wave from the quake, traveling at the speed of sound through the Earth, was detected by seismometers around the world, but while each seismic station knew there had been a major earthquake, they did not immediately know where. All they knew was the time when the shock waves arrived at their seismometer.

Actually, two shocks are recorded: the P-wave, or compression wave, that travels through the Earth, and an S-wave that travels along the surface like a wave on the ocean. The P-wave travels faster. From the separation between the P and S waves, the distance from the seismometer to the epicenter can be calculated. If the distance from three widely separated stations is known, scientists can pinpoint the location of the quake.

The most modern seismic stations are located around the Pacific Ocean: Japan, Hawaii, and the west coast of the Americas in particular. The rim of the Pacific has a history of severe volcanic eruptions, earthquakes, and tsunamis. The seismic stations are monitored twenty-four hours a day, but precious minutes were lost in communicating between stations and doing the calculations. By the time it was determined that it was one of the most powerful quakes ever recorded and the epicenter was in Indian Ocean, the tsunami was most of the way to Banda Aceh. Even then there might have been time to warn people in low-lying areas—anyone with a map could see where it would hit—but no one knew how to contact local officials in these largely Third-World regions. Nor would most local officials have had the means to spread the alarm.

The sad reality was that in the regions of greatest devastation, the tsunami struck shore after shore virtually without warning for hours after the earthquake had been located.

PROTECTION

Even as the nations of the world rushed relief supplies, medical assistance, and construction teams to the areas devastated by the tsunami, planning was underway to prevent another such disaster. Science is nowhere near being able to predict earthquakes, much less prevent them, but modern communications can spread a tsunami warning at the speed of light.

There is always concern that even a severe quake may only be a prelude to a still larger one. The first step, therefore, was to install unmanned, solar-powered warning buoys that sense the passage of a tsunami and automatically sound the warning to coastal areas. Such warning devices are already in use in some places around the Pacific. They include such technologies as solar-electric panels, satellite communications, the Global Positioning System, and mobile microwave telephones that did not exist even a decade ago.

The next step, still underway, is to tie all seismic stations into a central computer that will automatically collect and analyze seismic signals, carry out the calculations, send warnings to threatened areas, and inform governments—all without human involvement. Efforts will be concentrated most heavily in regions of high elastic stress in the Earth's crust, where tectonic movement is most likely.

This is the twenty-first Century. No longer must we submit meekly to the blind forces of nature. If all of humanity were to crowd into every place of worship on the planet to pray to their gods that Earth be spared another such disaster, yet will the movement of the Earth's crust continue without the pause of a single atom. But we can turn to science to lessen the suffering caused by that movement.

CHAPTER SEVEN

THE NEW AGE

In which anything goes

Adam Dreamhealer became a millionaire before his twentieth birthday. A college student, whose real name is kept secret to protect his privacy, Adam is the author of several profitable books, and his "seminars" in a five-hundred-seat auditorium are sold out weeks in advance. Adam describes himself as an "energy-healer." On stage he goes into a trance-like state in which he projects his mind into the bodies of cancer victims to "see" their cancer. Without touching them, Adam eliminates their cancer using only the power of his mind. He calls the technique "quantum-holography."

He will also treat people privately—even if they are in a distant city. These personalized remote sessions, of course, are much more expensive than the "seminars." Adam readily admits that his treatments don't always work the first time and may need to be repeated several times. The patient must pay for each session, but who's complaining if it cures their cancer? But does it cure their cancer?

Adam explains that he was given this remarkable power on a visit to Nootka Island near Vancouver when he was fifteen. On the island he encountered a strange four-foot-tall blackbird that communicated with him telepathically, downloading all of the world's knowledge into his brain. It's anybody's guess how

a four-foot-tall blackbird had acquired all the world's knowledge, or why it picked Adam to be a repository.

I first learned about Adam from an ABC News producer
who was working on a story for the television news magazine
Primetime. He showed me several videos of Adam's "seminars"
taken by ABC. Because Adam insists on working with the lights
dimmed, they were taken with an infrared camera. The ghostly
green of the infrared-detector images heightened the supernatural impression. Adam is seen using his hands as though he is
rearranging things that the rest of us can't see. Presumably he's
making adjustments to a quantum hologram of the patient. He
must have borrowed his quantum hologram from Tom Cruise,
who used it in the futuristic Steven Spielberg thriller *Minority
Report*. The big bird notwithstanding, there is nothing to suggest that Adam has any inkling of what a hologram is, much
less quantum physics.

ABC flew me to New York to talk about it. The *Primetime*
producer wanted to know what information would be needed
to evaluate Adam's claims. "First you should ask for test results
to confirm that the technique actually works," I told him. "At
a minimum, meaningful tests would require that the patient's
cancer be independently verified by qualified medical experts
before the treatment. That usually means a biopsy. The same
experts should examine the patient after the treatment to see if
there has been any change." Energy-healers build their resumes
by curing people of cancers they never had in the first place.

"There have been no tests, and no biopsies," the producer
confessed. "In that case," I told him, "there is nothing to evaluate. It would be irresponsible of ABC to give Adam free exposure on nationwide television without solid test results."

In the end, of course, ABC News went ahead, devoting a full
hour of *Primetime* to Adam Dreamhealer. After all, tests take
time and television runs on a schedule. Nevertheless, by exposing a "healer" who preys on victims of cancer as fraudulent,
ABC News imagined it was performing an important public
service. It's not that simple. Of the millions of people who

viewed *Primetime*, most had never before heard of Adam Dreamhealer. Adam is not running for political office so he doesn't have to convince them all of his power, or even a majority. Far from it. If only one viewer in ten thousand thinks there might be something to his story, Adam stands to take in another million dollars. I expect he would gladly pay ABC for the privilege of being exposed on *Primetime*.

In the absence of any test results, there is no reason to believe that Adam has the power to cure cancer. The only interesting question is, why anyone would imagine that he could? What would cause an otherwise rational person to accept Adam's preposterous story of a big blackbird telepathically infusing him with the power to cure cancer?

"When a man knows he is to be hanged in a fortnight," Samuel Johnson said in 1775, "it concentrates his mind wonderfully." With all due respect to Dr. Johnson, I find it more often has the opposite effect. People who are suffering chronic pain or believe they have a terminal illness will grasp at anything. The more hopeless their condition, the more likely people are to buy snake oil or fall to their knees before imaginary gods. They may even resort to "quantum holography" and telepathic blackbirds. They have little to lose. But as we will see below, even among those who would seem to have everything, irrational beliefs are not uncommon.

In the previous chapters we examined ancient superstitions that are fundamental to many of the world's religions. Notwithstanding the absence of any scientific support for religious superstitions, the overwhelming majority of people accept the superstitious beliefs of their own religion without question. Why wouldn't they? In this difficult world we have little choice but to rely on the word of people we trust. Religious superstitions don't come just from the pulpit; the most trusted and admired people in our society—parents, teachers, political leaders, even sports heroes and entertainers—often proclaim their religious convictions publicly. After all, religious belief is generally regarded as a virtue. In Bible-Belt America, children may be in college before they discover that nonbelief is an option.

Adam Dreamhealer never invokes God or angels, preferring instead to identify a big telepathic blackbird as the supernatural source of his power. This is New Age spirituality; it avoids direct competition with the more conventional religious miracles of the faith healers. There's plenty of gravy here for everyone, so why should a New Age energy-healer squabble with faith healers? Adam's appeal is primarily to the alienated, who feel that God and science have both failed them. The resort to utter nonsense may be due more to desperation than to weakness of character.

To understand the powerful appeal of New Age mysticism, we must examine how the brain forms beliefs.

THE AMYGDALAE

From the moment of birth the human brain is busily processing input from the senses to generate beliefs about what is and what isn't so in the strange world in which the newborn finds itself. Having few beliefs to contradict new information, the young are particularly open to new beliefs. They tend to accept everything initially, but because their beliefs have not yet become enmeshed in a matrix of related beliefs, children can also cast beliefs off almost as easily as they are adopted.

People keep adding to and amending their personal guidebook to life on planet Earth throughout life, and inevitably conflicts arise between new sensory input and existing beliefs that must somehow be reconciled. The number of conflicts keeps growing as we go through life, making it more difficult to add new beliefs. Indoctrination in a particular set of beliefs is therefore most successful when it's started early in life, frequently reinforced, and linked to a well-defined worldview. "Give me the boy until he is seven," Jesuits say, "and I will show you the man."

A belief starts with sensory input, which is routed through the thalamus, a small subsection deep within the brain. The thalamus normally directs sensory input to the sensory cortex, which analyses it and assigns an importance level. This information is then passed on to the amygdalae, the almond-shaped structures in the temporal lobes that generate an emotional response. The amygdalae are the seat of our Personal Guidebook to Life on Planet Earth.

A belief begins when the sensory cortex makes an association between two events, such as a particularly high tide coinciding with a full moon directly overhead. The next time you're on the beach at midnight under a full moon, your brain is primed to expect another high tide—but only if your brain retains the memory of the earlier high tide under a full moon. It has, after all, been some multiple of twenty-eight days since you could have last observed the coincidence, and memories fade with time. If the coincidence is repeated before the memory is lost, however, the memory may become a belief. Repetition, as every teacher knows, is the key to learning.

How long our brain retains a memory depends on the significance assigned to the event by the sensory cortex. The significance is equated to the level of arousal hormones in the bloodstream. One can imagine midnight encounters on a warm beach beneath a full moon that would lead to a very high state of emotional arousal. Indeed, just reading these words may lead you to imagine such an encounter. The response of the amygdalae to that thought would be to instruct the hypothalamus to release various arousal hormones into your bloodstream, mimicking the cocktail that led to the memory. As a result, your blood pressure and heart rate will be elevated. A very ancient section of the brain, the hypothalamus (literally "below the thalamus") is responsible for controlling the flow of hormones on instructions from the amygdalae. We are all manipulated by our hormones, depending on the beliefs and memories stored in the amygdalae.

The advent of language opened a powerful new channel for the creation of beliefs. Language makes vicarious experience the dominant source of beliefs, overwhelming personal experience. The power of language was greatly amplified by the invention of writing, and is further amplified by every new advance in communications, from the printing press to the BlackBerry. Beliefs can now spread around the world in the twinkling of a computer chip. Unfortunately, that which allows us to learn from others also exposes us to manipulation by them.

If the arousal level is high enough, the thalamus may choose to simply bypass the sensory cortex and route the sensory input directly to the amygdalae. The thalamus hasn't a clue as to which sensory input is causing the hormone rush, so it simply sends everything along. That's why we remember all the details of where we were and what we were doing when we heard the news about the 9/11 attack on the World Trade Center.

Such events are also the origin of personal superstitions, the little rituals we all perform to re-create the conditions we associate with some moment of high gratification, or to avoid those things we associate with unpleasantness. An athlete might always eat the same breakfast before a game, or you might wear your lucky tie to an important meeting. This is imitative or sympathetic magic. Unless we become truly obsessed by them, such personal superstitions are harmless, and at times may even be beneficial by raising a person's confidence level.

SIGNAL-TO-NOISE RATIO

The processing of vast amounts of sensory information to form beliefs about the world goes on during every waking moment. Over time, these beliefs define who we are, but they are often flawed. All sensory inputs carry some level of "noise" that degrades the quality of the information: there may have been traffic noise in the background, for example, or it was dusk and the light was dim, or perhaps there were distractions. All these things are noise. In attempting to attach meaning to sensory inputs that are obscured by noise, the brain tries to help by filling in the picture with details borrowed from memory—including memories that may themselves be flawed.

As a graduate student fifty years ago I worked summers for a university laboratory doing sonar research for the navy. It had become apparent during World War II that there is a large variation in the ability of sonar operators to make sense of the clutter of sounds picked up by the hydrophones of a submarine. Some operators could identify the faint sound of a distant ship's screw even in the presence of much louder background noises. The difference in operator ability went far beyond the results of standard hearing tests. Was this something that could be taught to operators? Or if not, could we screen for this ability?

As a first step, an experiment was conducted in which sonar operators listened on their headphones to a background of random noise. A string of spoken words was then superimposed on the noise background. The operator's task was to write down what they heard. The spoken words would be repeated with increasing volume until the operator could make them out above the noise. It was expected that what the operators heard would initially be garbled, but would improve each time the volume level of the spoken words was increased relative to the background.

To get a good baseline, the background noise was kept on the headphones for some period of time before the spoken line was superimposed. No one, however, thought to inform the operators of this dead period. The result was unexpected. Often the operators began writing down words they "heard" almost immediately—before there were any words to hear. Their brains were struggling to make sense of the random background noise. It was a sort of audio Rorschach test, offering a glimpse into the mind of the operator.

It was a sobering revelation: there are pages in everyone's Personal Guidebook to Life on Planet Earth that are cobbled together from noisy and incomplete sensory inputs. Gaps are filled in with scraps borrowed from other pages. Everything seems to be more or less in the right place, but like Dr. Frankenstein's monster, parts have been taken from different bodies, and the collective result can be scary.

ASK YOUR AMYGDALAE

I was jogging along the trail beside Northwest Branch one evening at dusk, when I spotted a large animal crossing into the woods farther up the trail. That far away in the fading light, I thought it looked like a bear. I felt the tingle of a slight adrenalin surge. A bear would be exciting; one had been captured in these woods, but that was years ago. The animal I saw looked to be about the size of the pygmy rhino I had seen on the morning news, but pygmy rhinos are confined to one small Indonesian island. I might have thought of Bigfoot, except I know Bigfoot is pure fantasy. Or could I have seen a mugger taking up a position behind a tree to pounce on an unwary jogger? More likely, it was just a large dog.

My brain was doing what brains do when confronted with noisy and incomplete sensory input. It was trying to reconcile the noisy image that briefly registered on my retina with all the other stuff I keep stored in my Personal Guidebook to Life on Planet Earth. Because the sighting was given a "significant" rating by my sensory cortex, the amygdalae were instructing the hypothalamus to release a cocktail of hormones that would determine my reaction. Which hormones the amygdalae call for depends on the anxieties and prejudices they find among my beliefs. If caution dominates, I will slow down or turn around. If curiosity wins, I will speed up to get a better look at whatever it is before it gets away.

It's up to the amygdalae. The brain, of course, operates electrochemically rather than electromagnetically, so it's not as fast as Google. Nevertheless, the amygdalae come up with a surprising number of hits in a pretty short time. Like Google, however, you can't assume that all the information is reliable or relevant.

Jogging alone through the woods as darkness approaches is not recommended. Dangerous or not someone from another culture might have reacted quite differently to the sight of a dark figure crossing the trail at dusk. An Inuit on a trail above the Arctic Circle at dusk might think he had seen an Amarok, a giant wolf in Inuit mythology that devours anyone foolish enough to be hunting alone when darkness falls. Perhaps we need a similar myth for joggers.

In the Middle Ages, a Christian might have thought it was a demon. Satan's demons were everywhere back then, roaming the countryside at dusk looking for human souls to take back to hell. Such scary myths were no doubt invented to discourage dangerous or improper behavior, and were usually incorporated into religious teaching. Today, however, science scoffs at notions of Amaroks or demons in the dusk, and warns that it's exposure to unscreened ultraviolet radiation from the midday sun that we should fear. The difference is that science has done the research to back up its warning.

BELIEVING IN BELIEF

But what of those who are grounded in neither science nor religion? How do they decide what to believe? Simple—they join the New Age revolution and believe in everything. Beginning in the 1980s, the New Age movement embraced spiritualism, reincarnation, channeling, mediums, holistic healing, astrology, crystals, pyramid power, and more. Lacking guidance from a sacred book or tradition, belief itself becomes the unifying principle behind the New Age.

When I first heard in December of 2006 that a book called *The Secret* by Rhonda Byrne was at the top of the *New York Times* best-seller list, I was puzzled. I follow the book-review section of the *Times* and the *Washington Post* pretty closely each week, but I hadn't noticed a book listed with that title under either fiction or nonfiction. Nor had I ever heard of Rhonda Byrne.

I had forgotten "advice," a category created in the 1990s when New Age books by Deepak Chopra with wacky titles like

The Quantum Alternative to Growing Old began dominating the nonfiction list. I'm pretty sure there is only one alternative to growing old, and I don't recommend it. Nonetheless, Chopra once had four books in the nonfiction top-10 at the same time. The fact that Chopra's pseudoscientific New Age blather sells at all is a sad commentary on reading tastes, but we don't burn books anymore, even terrible books. However, we do segregate them. It's not a perfect solution.

A couple of weeks later, a reporter called to ask what scientists thought about *The Secret*. "Why," I asked, "is it a science book?" "No, no," he replied, obviously shocked that I was so poorly informed about a book that outsold the latest Harry Potter adventure, "but it does quote a lot of physicists." In fact, I was unable to find a single physicist I knew who had ever heard of the book.

In taking over the number-one spot in the advice category, *The Secret* replaced Gary Trudeau's *Natural Cures "They" Don't Want You to Know About*. Trudeau, who never finished grade school, is a forty-four-year-old ex-convict and infomercial guru. He has been fined $2 million by the FTC for dishonest sales practices and barred from selling on television infomercials, but under the First Amendment he can still write books. He wears his criminal convictions as badges of honor—proof that the establishment is trying to silence him.

In addition to Trudeau's quack medicine, the advice category is where they put all the new diet plans, celebrity tell-alls, and self-help sex therapy. It's also where they put the New Age books. The advice category can best be described as "books for people who watch daytime television." *The Secret* fits perfectly.

OPRAH IS "THE SECRET"

In the preface to her thin little volume, Rhonda Byrne makes the incredible promise that "as you learn The Secret, you will come to know how you can have, be, or do anything you want."

She doesn't keep you waiting. In the first chapter, "The Se-cret Revealed," the reader learns that "quantum physicists tell us the entire Universe emerged from thought." It doesn't say who these quantum physicists are, or who was doing the think-ing that created the universe. Throughout the book, however, there are references to the power of thought to become things.

At the end of the chapter there is a summary of The Secret. Had they known there would be a summary, readers could have spared themselves the preceding twenty-four pages of tired self-help clichés contributed by New Age gurus. They don't add much anyway, beyond showing that this is not just one person's delusion. The main points:

- The Great Secret of Life is the law of attraction. When you think a thought, you are also attracting like thoughts to you.
- Your current thoughts are creating your future life. What you think about the most will appear as your life.
- Your thoughts become things.

That's it—that's The Secret. Whether you want to get rich or get laid, you just have to want it enough, and not let those negative thoughts creep in. The main purpose in life, reinforced on almost every page, is to satisfy your greed by attracting wealth to yourself. You're poor? You should have thought of yourself as rich.

It's foolish, but it's also terribly cruel. You've got terminal cancer? You must have attracted the cancer to yourself by fear-ing cancer. Your child has asthma? It's because you failed to think of him as healthy.

The great champion of *The Secret*, who single-handedly made it a runaway best-seller, is Oprah Winfrey, the queen of day-time television. Oprah sees herself as the embodiment of the book's promise: She craved wealth, power, fame, and sex, and was absolutely convinced she would have it. She now has it all. And by featuring *The Secret* twice on her popular daytime talk show, Oprah guaranteed it would be a huge financial success. I mean, isn't that how The Secret works?

THE POSITIVE PREACHER

But is any of this new? It all sounded so familiar. In particular, the last bullet of Rhonda Bryne's summary: Your thoughts become things. I seemed to remember trying, years ago, to figure out whether that was meant literally or metaphorically. I searched out a copy of Norman Vincent Peale's 1952 best-seller, *The Power of Positive Thinking*, a book that stayed on the *New York Times* best-seller list for 186 consecutive weeks and sold 7 million copies. Yes, there it was on page 169: "Thoughts are things." *The Secret* is a New Age replay of *The Power of Positive Thinking*.

Raised as a Methodist, and ordained as a minister in 1922, Norman Vincent Peale later changed his affiliation to the Reformed Church in America, and became one of New York City's most famous preachers. For fifty-four years he hosted a weekly radio program, *The Art of Living*. In 1984 President Ronald Reagan awarded Peale the Presidential Medal of Freedom, the highest civilian honor in the United States, for contributions to the field of theology.

Peale's theology, however, is less concerned with salvation and worship, which he felt produced little result, than with persuading people to apply his "positive thinking" techniques to "channel God's power," thus achieving success in everything a person undertakes—especially becoming rich. This requires an intense program of self-hypnosis, and the total repression of any negative thoughts.

Peale was New Age before New Age was invented. In *The Power of Positive Thinking*, he claimed that scientific experts, never identified by name, supported his philosophy and had verified the benefits of his positive-thinking technique. In fact, Peale's self-hypnosis technique was heavily criticized by mental health experts, who warned that it was dangerous. Critics denounced him as a con man and a fraud. As a minister, however, Peale was spared from any requirement to prove his assertions.

Today, Peale's methods do not seem very different from the meditation methods of Dr. Herbert Benson's "relaxation response" discussed in chapter 3. Benson, however, whom I would place on the fringe of the New Age movement, claims only health benefits, while Peale promised "success," by which he means "money."

By following his positive-thinking methods, Peale insisted, you cause positive things to happen, while negative thoughts cause negative things to happen. Fifty years later, that is precisely what is being claimed in *The Secret*, yet nowhere is Norman Vincent Peale mentioned.

THE QUANTUM PLOY

The lack of any sacred text to connect the seemingly unrelated beliefs and practices that make up the New Age movement might seem to put it at a disadvantage with respect to organized religion. Instead of religious doctrine, however, the New Age movement claims to find confirmation in science, specifically the science of quantum physics. It's a clever strategy, relying on the public's unfamiliarity with the mathematical foundations of quantum theory.

The Secret includes brief contributions from several renegade PhD physicists who also appear in the deplorable film *What the (bleep) Do We Know?* These are people who have made little contribution to science, but who seem to enjoy misleading an audience with special effects meant to show how weird quantum-physics effects would seem if they carried over to the scale of the human body. In fact, the laws of quantum physics smoothly transition to the familiar laws of classical physics as the number of atoms is increased.

Quantum physics is one of the greatest intellectual accomplishments of our species, but it is still science in the making.

CHAPTER EIGHT

SCHRÖDINGER'S GRAVE

In which quantum mysticism is found to be superstition

For twenty-eight years, the cramped little laboratory in the basement of an engineering building on the Princeton University campus was famous around the world for rigorous scientific studies of the influence of human consciousness on machines. On February 10, 2007, however, Robert G. Jahn, founder of the Princeton Engineering Anomalies Research Laboratory, abruptly announced that the lab would close its doors forever at the end of the month.

At seventy-six, Jahn had been a Princeton man for his entire adult life. An exceptional student in the class of 1951, he graduated with highest honors in engineering physics. He once described his student years as a "period of high church" for physicists. If so, Princeton, New Jersey, was the Holy City. Drawn by the presence of Albert Einstein at the Center for Advanced Study, the great thinkers who led the twentieth century revolution in physics, including Niels Bohr and Werner Heisenberg, traveled to Princeton and lectured at the university.

Jahn thrived in this stimulating atmosphere, remaining at Princeton for a doctoral degree and eventually joining the faculty in 1962 as an assistant professor of aeronautical engineering. Popular among the students for his unconventional views and energetic lectures, Jahn became a bridge between the student body and the university administration during the unrest over the Vietnam War. He helped to keep Princeton relatively calm at a time when chaos ruled at many American colleges. The university administration began taking notice of this talented young engineering professor. He rose quickly through the ranks, in 1971 becoming dean of the engineering school, which flourished under his direction. But administration bored Robert Jahn. Since his undergraduate days, it had been the puzzling developments in quantum physics that fascinated him.

You breathed quantum physics at Princeton.

MAKING WAVES

In the summer of 2000, I was invited to speak at the Alpbach European Forum, a two-week conference on science, the arts, and politics held each August in the beautiful Austrian village of Alpbach in the Tyrolean Alps. I had read somewhere that Erwin Schrödinger (1887–1961), the father of modern quantum theory, was buried in a churchyard in Alpbach. In view of his unconventional life style, it seemed ironic that his final resting place would be in a churchyard—among other things, Schrödinger's domestic arrangement was a ménage à trois. The Catholic church in Alpbach was directly across the winding cobblestone road that ran by the small alpine-style hotel in which I was staying with my wife and oldest son.

We could find no tourist information to help us out, so the three of us split up and began examining every grave marker in the little churchyard. It did not take long to locate a marker for Erwin Rudolf Josef Alexander Schrödinger. The only inscription beneath his name was a partial differential equation, recognizable to every physicist as "Schrödinger's equation." It is the starting point for almost every quantum mechanical calculation, and has correctly predicted the outcome of countless experiments, leading finally to the miracles of modern electronics technology. Even Heisenberg's "uncertainty principle," one of the cornerstones of quantum mechanics, emerges naturally from Schrödinger's "wave equation."

HEISENBERG WAS CERTAIN

In an earlier book, *Voodoo Science*, I used the example of clocking the speed of an automobile to illustrate the classic dilemma of measurement. You could set up two pylons on the side of the road a known distance apart. An observer at pylon one presses a button that starts a clock running when the car passes; a second observer presses a button that stops the clock when the car passes pylon two. Divide the distance between the pylons by the time on the clock, and you now have a measure of the car's speed.

Each time you make the measurement, however, you will get a slightly different result. As in all measurements, there are sources of "noise" having to do with the accuracy with which distance or time is measured—the reaction time of the observers, for example. The noise could be reduced by replacing the observers with automatic photocells, measuring the distance between the pylons with an interferometer, and replacing the clock with an atomic clock. Most simply, you could reduce the relative contribution of noise by simply moving the pylons farther apart.

The farther you move the pylons apart to improve the relative accuracy, however, the less certain you can be about where the car is when it is traveling between the pylons. If asked, your answer would have to be "between the pylons."

This trade-off is the classic dilemma of measurement. It had always been assumed that with better design and sufficient resources, you would be able to reduce the uncertainties as far as you wish. It was time for one of the greatest scientific insights in history. It came from a young German physicist still in his twenties.

Werner Heisenberg proposed that the Planck constant—the ratio of the energy of one quantum of radiation to its frequency—defines a fundamental limit on how accurately you can simultaneously know both the position and momentum of an object. Heisenberg pointed out that in observing the smallest parts of the world, the act of observation alters the thing observed. The two monumental scientific theories that defined the twentieth century, relativity and quantum mechanics, both made the observer part of the physics. In 1932 Heisenberg was awarded the Nobel Prize in physics for "the creation of quantum mechanics." The world would never be the same again.

UNCERTAINTY

A year after Heisenberg was awarded the Nobel Prize, Erwin Schrödinger shared the prize with Paul Dirac for "the discovery of new productive forms of quantum theory." Schrödinger had earlier moved from Vienna to Berlin to occupy the position that had been held by Max Planck. Berlin was at that time the leading center of science in the world, and it was there that Schrödinger developed his wave equation for which he was awarded the Nobel Prize. But 1933 was also the year that Hitler came to power in Germany, and Schrödinger, appalled by anti-Semitism under the Nazis, decided he could not remain in Germany. The Nobel Prize has a way of opening all doors. He received his Nobel Prize not in Germany but at Oxford University, infuriating the Nazis.

In 1936 he was offered a position at the University of Graz in his native Austria. In spite of strong misgivings about of the worsening political climate in Europe, he could not resist an opportunity to return to Austria. Two years later, however, Germany annexed Austria and Schrödinger found himself in serious trouble. His departure from Berlin just before being awarded the 1933 Nobel Prize had embarrassed the Nazis. He managed to escape through Italy, however, and eventually ended up at the new Institute for Advanced Studies in Dublin, where he would become director and remain until his retirement in 1955, when he returned to Austria.

Generations of physics students equate quantum physics with Schrödinger's wave equation, treating the wave function as a probability distribution. The amplitude of the wave function at any point represents the probability of finding an electron there. The solution to Schrödinger's equation for an electron in some sort of potential well is an inevitable final exam problem in elementary quantum mechanics.

Now suppose that you actually detect the electron with your instruments. There is no longer any uncertainty about its location. The act of observing the electron is said to "collapse" the wave function to that point. To some scientists the collapse of the wave function made it seem as if the conscious act of observation actually created the thing observed, turning a fuzzy probability function into a thing—even though Schrödinger himself had ridiculed this interpretation.

Everyone agreed that the Schrödinger equation worked, and there were millions of important calculations waiting to be done. It was a time of great opportunity, translating classical descriptions of nature into the language of quantum physics—even if there was some disagreement about how to explain it. Why not just agree that nature behaves as if reality depends on the conscious act of an observer and get on with it? Inevitably however, scientists began to omit the phrase "as if" from their discussions. Why bother, everything was working fine?

Some took it much farther, arguing that since events on an atomic scale are affected by the act of observation, and since everything in the universe is made of atoms, we should not be surprised to find our thoughts influencing events on the macroscopic scale in which our lives are lived. Those with a spiritual bent began talking about "universal consciousness."

This was a godsend for the paranormal community. It provided scientific cover for every New Age fantasy from telepathy to feng shui. New Age technobabble was sprinkled with "quantum non-locality," "entanglement," and "collapsing" wave functions. The CIA would spend millions on "remote viewing," and

Rhonda Bryne's *The Secret* would become a runaway bestseller. To the question, "How can that be?" the standard answer became "quantum mechanics."

COLLAPSING REALITY

Many scientists seemed to enjoy their status as ordained quantum priests presiding over mysterious rituals in a strange language, rather like conducting mass in Latin. To strip away some of the vestments and see what's underneath, let's do a simple thought experiment.

We put a white ball and a black ball in separate but identical boxes. The boxes are then shuffled; I put one in my pocket and you take the other. We then climb into our respective spaceships and leave Earth headed in opposite directions. I have no way of knowing whether my box contains the white ball or the black ball. In the language of quantum mechanics, a wave function for the white ball is half in my box and half in yours on the other side of the galaxy. The same is true of the wave function of the black ball. If I don't peek, there is only a "potential" ball inside the box.

Some day, when my curiosity gets the best of me, I will open my box. Perhaps I will find a white ball inside. In quantum-speak, the act of making the observation would be said to have created the white ball by "collapsing" the white ball's wave function—including the 50% in your box halfway across the galaxy. Had information traveled superluminally (faster than light) through a universal consciousness field?

I can't prove it's not so—in the language of philosophers, it's not falsifiable—but it doesn't seem to be a very useful concept.

RANDOM EVENTS?

One of those who thought quantum mechanics implied some sort of universal consciousness was Robert Jahn at Princeton, and he firmly believed it to be the responsibility of scientists to find out. If true, it would profoundly alter our understanding of reality.

Another who thought so was German-born physicist and parapsychologist Helmut Schmidt at the Rhine Research Center's Institute for Parapsychology in Durham, North Carolina. Schmidt initiated research into the effects of human consciousness on machines called random number generators (RNGs) in the 1970s. A random number generator can be thought of as a device that flips a coin for you over and over, keeping track of the heads and tails. RNGs have found use as controls in many experiments involving statistical analysis.

Actually flipping a coin enough times to get good statistics would be rather time consuming. Schmidt's device, however, was electronic, switching randomly between a red and a green light. RNGs normally do this by triggering on "white" electrical noise. "White noise" literally means the spectrum is of equal intensity at every frequency. Any noise spike above a preset level would switch the color of light. Familiar sources of white noise are the hiss from a radio that is not tuned to a station and the sound of rushing water. A subject would attempt to influence with his mind which color was lit more often.

Whether you can actually make a machine that is truly random is disputed by some experts, but even if that's so, Schmidt felt he could control for it by having his subjects alternate between periods of thinking green and thinking red. The electronic RNG allowed Schmidt to accumulate statistically significant results relatively quickly.

In hundreds of trials, Schmidt reported success rates of 1% to 2% above what would be expected if the RNG was not influenced by the subject's thoughts. One extra "heads" out of a hundred coin tosses may not sound like much, but if the mind of the subject was exerting any influence, however small, it would be a revolutionary discovery—if it was real.

Psychokinesis, or "telekinesis" as it was generally called in the 1970s, captured the public imagination. You will recall from chapter 3 that Israeli psychic Uri Geller baffled two physicists,

Harold Puttoff and Russell Targ, at the Stanford Research Institute with a simple parlor trick in which he appeared to bend spoons with the power of his mind. Brian De Palma's 1976 film *Carrie*, about an angry teenage girl's psychokinetic rampage, was a huge box-office success. There was even a television game show on NBC called *Blank Check* that was supposed to reward contestants for their ESP powers. It folded after only a couple of episodes because none of the contestants, all of whom imagined themselves as having great psychic power, could outperform a coin toss.

Because Helmut Schmidt's random-number-generator experiments in Durham had all the trappings of a serious scientific study, they were taken seriously by people who probably should have known better.

MIND GAMES

There was, however, a far more serious side to the ESP fad of the 1970s. Fifteen hundred miles away from Durham at the Los Alamos National Laboratory in New Mexico, those responsible for ensuring the safety of America's vast stockpile of nuclear bombs held urgent top-secret meetings to discuss Schmidt's findings. Engineers calculated the force that would be needed, and the distance over which it would have to operate, to set off a nuclear bomb. Considering the consequences, the amount of energy it would take to trigger a warhead seemed frighteningly small. In the design of nuclear weapons the emphasis had been on ensuring that there was no way to apply such a force externally, but could the mind reach inside the bomb?

Two hundred and fifty thousand miles away on the Moon, astronaut Edgar Mitchell, excited by Schmidt's results, conducted private ESP experiments with friends on Earth. The experiments consisted of Mitchell concentrating on one of five different cards and his psychic friends back on Earth trying to tell which one. The result according to Mitchell was that ESP worked about as well across 250,000 miles of empty space as it does with someone in the same room. Actually, I'm prepared to believe it would work exactly as well. Believers take this as evidence of "quantum non-locality."

Three hundred and eighty miles away at Princeton University, a student proposed, as her undergraduate thesis project, building a random number generator similar to Schmidt's for the study of psychokinesis. She asked Robert Jahn, by then dean of the engineering school, if he would supervise her project. It would become his life's work.

PEAR

In 1979 Robert Jahn announced the formation of the Princeton Engineering Anomalies Research (PEAR) lab. The first project of the new lab would be to replicate Schmidt's random-number-generator experiments. In the years that followed, the PEAR lab would find a small positive result in millions of trials using a wide variety of random devices.

There were "random-walk" machines, battery operated toys that randomly changed direction. The subject would mentally urge the random-walk machine to go in a particular direction. Although the path taken by the machine might appear random to an observer, the automated machinery that tracked the device always seemed to compute with great certainty that the motion of the device had been influenced by the thoughts of the subject.

There were experiments with water fountains, in which water droplets are randomly generated by the fluid stream. The subject would urge the fountain to kick a drop ever higher. Again, the automated analysis would somehow calculate astronomical odds against the outcome being mere chance.

Was fraud involved? It can't be ruled out. Most of the PEAR trials were conducted by the staff. Life is better in any organization if the boss is happy, and the staff is usually quick to figure out what it takes to make the boss happy. Fraud, of course, implies intention. Unconscious bias, however, is a far more serious possibility.

Although PEAR seemed to have taken reasonable measures to eliminate investigator bias, the basic design of the experiments remained unchanged for twenty-eight years. The philosophy of the lab was that the more times they repeated the trial, the more statistical power the conclusion would have, so they kept it up year after year. Up to a point that's a reasonable assumption. Unfortunately, repetition does not average out systematic errors, either mechanical or human.

Even flipping a coin, since a coin is not perfectly symmetric, might be expected to differ between heads and tails, but it would take a great many flips for the tiny difference to show up. With enough repetitions, seeming insignificant flaws in the design of any random device begin to emerge from the results as the statistical noise diminishes.

In a randomized double-blind version of the PEAR trials, the decision about which light, red or green, the subject would concentrate on might be made by a second RNG but would not be known to the person recording the results. Only after the trials were completed would the records be compared to find the number of hits. If the slight margin on which PEAR based its claims of psychokinesis were the result of experimenter bias, the margin would vanish. But, of course, a double-blind version was never tried—or at least never reported.

Physicists rarely consider doing double-blind experiments, believing they are useful only in subjective medical trials to get around the placebo effect. However, I find numerous cases where a double-blind physics experiment would have spared researchers subsequent embarrassment.

Several times over the years I recommended that PEAR attempt an entirely different demonstration of psychokinesis. Instead of statistically analyzing the output of random number generators, why not use a state-of-the-art microbalance to directly measure the psychokinetic force exerted by the mind? Modern microbalances have sensitivities in the pico-newton range. Simply zero the microbalance and then attempt to unbalance it by the force of thought. If it moves, it would not only be the first direct demonstration of psychokinesis, it would provide a direct physical measurement of the force exerted by thought. Alas, microbalances are never used in these experiments for the simple reason that they stubbornly refuse to budge, no matter how hard the subject concentrates. Indeed, even if several people concentrate in unison, nothing happens. If every person on Earth had joined in the effort, I am quite sure there would still have been no effect. No amount of wishing it were otherwise can change that.

GLOBAL DISASTERS

After almost twenty years of random-number-generator studies at the PEAR laboratory, the work expanded into an international collaboration in 1998. The Global Consciousness Project involved a network of sixty-five random number generators located around the world. The director of the project was Roger Nelson, a parapsychologist who had joined the PEAR team in 1980 and had conducted many of the RNG trials himself.

It was a major change of direction. The focus of PEAR for twenty years had been on the power of thought to control the output of an RNG. But if RNGs are affected by thoughts directed at them by the subject, could they also be responding to all the other traffic in the global consciousness field? There seemed to be no way to screen out the thought field.

During periods of high emotional arousal affecting large numbers of people around the globe, such as a major natural disaster, RNGs might be expected to exhibit unusual behavior. The Global Consciousness Project was formed to compare the output of all sixty-five RNGs in the network. But what constitutes anomalous behavior of a machine designed to give a random output? Deviations from randomness, of course. In other words, they would examine the output of the RNGs in the network to search for patterns.

Of course, the project found what it set out to find—and much more. They found "deviations from randomness" associated with such events as 9/11 and the funeral of Princess Di. Even more remarkably, there were deviations *before* major disasters such as the Christmas Tsunami in the Indian Ocean. You might think that any anomaly that occurred before a major event took place would be excluded—not at all. Not only were the RNGs responding to the shared emotions of the multitude, they anticipated the event that would produce the emotions. Random number generators, it must be concluded, are not only conscious, they are clairvoyant.

If any of this were true, it would dwarf all other human discoveries. The string of zeros and ones spewing from a random number generator might be telling us everything that will happen—if we could only break the code.

In abruptly announcing the closing of PEAR, Robert Jahn simply said it's time. "If people don't believe us after all the results we've produced," he told the *New York Times,* "then they never will." No one who knows Robert Jahn doubts his honesty or intelligence, but perhaps there was more to the decision to close PEAR than the weariness of its founder.

The Global Consciousness Project, which was becoming the most significant activity at PEAR, was not under Jahn's direct control. Perhaps, from a somewhat more detached perspective, the total absurdity of the Global Consciousness Project claims finally dawned on him. Was this what PEAR had become? Could he have been fooling himself all these years? It took millions of trials over a period of twenty-eight years to clearly expose the subtle flaw in the research—it was conducted by human beings.

We must ask how conscious a human observer must be to collapse a wave function? Could a chimpanzee, trained to make observations, collapse a wave function? What about a human who is no smarter than a chimpanzee? Robert Jahn did not stumble into the consciousness bog by himself. Other physicists have used "consciousness" in their descriptions. It's a sobering reminder that science has its own superstitions.

CHAPTER NINE

THE BARBARY DUCK

In which the body heals itself

As the flu season approached in the fall of 2004, the media, as they do each year, ran stories about the terrible flu pandemic of 1918 that killed 100 million people worldwide. The stories were accompanied by warnings from public health officials that it could happen again. The warnings are an annual ritual aimed at motivating the public to get their flu shots. There were troubling signs, however, that in 2004–2005 flu might be unusually severe.

Although it contributes to the death of thousands of humans every year, influenza is primarily a disease of birds. The flu virus mutates rapidly, and occasionally a mutation will enable a strain of bird flu to make the jump to another warm-blooded species. The 1918 flu pandemic apparently began as a bird virus. The rapid mutation of the flu virus makes it difficult to develop an effective vaccine.

To be effective, flu vaccine must incorporate a number of active strains, including the newest ones, and flu vaccine must be made anew each year. The United States contracted with Chiron Corporation in the United Kingdom for enough vaccine to cover demand in the winter of 2004–2005, even if it turned out to be a bad year for flu.

Then the unexpected happened. In October, British regulators forced Chiron to shut down its flu-production facility because of contamination problems. It was too late to cultivate more vaccine for the flu season that was just starting. The United States suddenly faced a critical shortage of vaccine.

Retiring Health and Human Services Secretary Tommy Thompson warned that the shortage put the United States at significant risk of another deadly flu pandemic. Instead of urging everyone to get a flu shot as they do most years, authorities began asking healthy people under fifty to forego vaccination. Nevertheless, lines snaked for blocks outside any facility that had vaccine. Supplies of the vaccine were often exhausted while people were still waiting in line. Those most at risk from flu, the elderly and those weakened by other illness, were least able to stand in line for hours and were generally allowed to go to the front of the line.

As the shortage grew, the *Wall Street Journal* ran a long article on flu shot alternatives. With flu vaccine in short supply, it must have seemed to the editors like the responsible thing to do. The first alternative on their list was FluMist. Available only by prescription, it is a live-virus vaccine administered by nasal spray. FluMist is highly effective, but because it uses a weakened form of live virus, it's not recommended for people over forty-nine or in poor health—the groups most at risk. The article also called for frequent hand washing, since flu spreads primarily from hand contact with surfaces that have been touched by others who have the virus. The *Wall Street Journal* also pointed out that if you're diagnosed with flu, your doctor can prescribe antiviral drugs, such amantadine, that should at least shorten the duration.

You can't argue with any of that. But the article included another alternative that drew groans from the scientific community. It listed oscillococcinum, a homeopathic medication, as an option. The only mild caveat was that "the homeopathic mechanism is questionable." But the homeopathic mechanism is not "questionable," it's nonexistent.

THE DILUTION LIMIT

Oscillococcinum sits on the pharmacy shelf beside other over-the-counter flu medications. These other medications do not claim to be able to cure or prevent flu, but rather to relieve symptoms such as nasal congestion and muscle aches, which they do with varying degrees of effectiveness. These other medications also list side effects such as drowsiness and dry mouth. But there are no side effects associated with oscillococcinum—there are no effects at all. People searching the flu shelf in a pharmacy for something to relieve their misery probably do not even notice the word "homeopathic" printed in small letters on the box. Many would have no idea what it means if they did. Most people believe any medicine sold in America must have been proven to be safe and effective. Unfortunately, that's not the case.

Congress has seen fit to enact certain exemptions to the pure food and drug laws. In particular, Senator Royal Copeland of New York, who was a homeopathic physician before entering the Senate, was the chief sponsor of the 1938 Food, Drug and Cosmetics Act. It included a provision explicitly exempting all homeopathic medications listed in the *Homeopathic Pharmacopoeia* from FDA oversight. That exemption is still on the books today. Copeland's justification for the exemption was quite simple: there is no way to confirm that a homeopathic preparation is what it claims to be. The effect of the exemption was to give homeopathy an edge over all the other snake oil on the market.

Oscillococcinum is made exclusively in France by Boiron Laboratories. Manufacturing begins with a substance allegedly prepared from the liver and heart of the Barbary duck. It's not clear why this particular species of wild duck was selected for the honor, but waterfowl are particularly susceptible to flu, and it's not inconceivable that something prepared from the internal organs of a duck could offer humans protection from the disease.

The next step in the Boiron process, however, is homeopathic dilution of the duck extract. The result, as we will see, is that oscillococcinum contains none of the substance derived from the organs of the duck. Not a single molecule.

As with any over-the-counter medication, the manufacturer is required to list the ingredients on the package. Boiron lists the active ingredient of oscillococcinum in Latin: *anas barbariae hepatis et cordis extractum*, "extract of the liver and heart of the Barbary duck." The concentration is given as 200CK HPUS. Few purchasers, I suspect, have any idea what that means. The "K" simply means that the oscillococcinum is diluted. The "C" means that the *initial* dilution is one part in a hundred. The "200" means that the dilution has been repeated sequentially 200 times. HPUS certifies that the ingredient is officially listed in the *Homeopathic Pharmacopoeia of the United States*—in other words, in accordance with the 1938 Copeland provision. Therefore oscillococcinum is exempt from FDA oversight. So what are you getting? You're getting ripped off.

Let's run the numbers: If you begin with a concentration of one part in a hundred and dilute it another one part in a hundred, you will have a concentration of one part in 10,000. Do it another time and you have one part in 1,000,000, and so on. Because all substances are made up of molecules, however, there is a limit. Suppose a point is reached at which only one molecule of oscillococcinum remains in the entire batch of medicine being prepared. That is the dilution limit. If it is diluted one more time, the odds would be 100 to 1 that not a single molecule of the substance remains. Depending on the size of the batch, the dilution limit will be reached after perhaps a dozen dilutions—and there are another 188 dilutions to go. "Dilution" beyond the dilution limit ceases to have any meaning. There is nothing to dilute.

Suppose we take the entire visible universe to be a "batch" of oscillococcinum. There are something like 10^{80} atoms in the visible universe, including all the stars in all the galaxies. That's a one followed by 80 zeroes. Suppose there is only one oscillococcinum molecule in the entire universe. What would be the homeopathic dilution of oscillococcinum in the universe? About 40C. To get more dilute than that we would need more universes—many billions more. Few homeopathic preparations claim a dilution of 200C, but 30C is quite standard in homeopathy. Even 30C, however, would exceed the dilution limit of an amount of oscillococcinum the size of the Earth. In plain words, homeopathic dilutions are completely meaningless. They far exceed the dilution limit. There is no medicine in the medicine.

If you point this out to homeopaths, they shrug their shoulders and acknowledge that the mechanism of homeopathy may not be fully understood, but millions of people around the world find it works. This includes Elizabeth II, the Queen of England, who has her own personal homeopath to provide her with a daily cocktail of homeopathic preparations. Somehow, according to homeopaths, the spiritual essence of the healing effect is retained even after the "active ingredient" is completely diluted away. In fact, they insist, repeating the dilutions even after the active substance is gone increases the potency. The water, they say, remembers.

I drink the water in Washington DC. It comes from the Potomac River, and I would prefer that the water not remember.

MONEY FOR NOTHING

Oscillococcinum is a $15 million-a-year business in the United States alone, and sells much more widely in Europe. A package of homeopathic oscillococcinum from Boiron sells for around $12, or about the price of a flu shot. The price represents the cost of guaranteeing that the medicine retains no trace of the active ingredient. Why, you may wonder, are millions of people around the world willing to pay twelve bucks for a guarantee that they are getting nothing? They are paying for the placebo effect—and placebos aren't free.

Oscillococcinum is advertised with the slogan "At the first sign of the flu, take oscillo." If someone takes oscillo at the first sneeze, and wakes up feeling fine the next morning, they will be inclined to believe that oscillo has spared them from a bout of the flu. The most likely explanation for reports of oscillococcinum's effectiveness is, therefore, simple misdiagnosis. In its early stages, flu can't be distinguished from numerous rhinovirus infections such as the common cold or allergic reactions to airborne pollen, mold spores, cat dandruff, and hundreds of other substances. Moreover, if someone does come down with a relatively mild strain of flu, they might conclude that oscillococcinum had spared them from a more serious bout, and still recommend it to others. Most of us are strongly influenced by testimonials coming from someone we know.

For most of human history, shared anecdotes were all people had to go on in seeking relief from illness. But no longer. The most important advance in medical research has been the randomized, placebo-controlled, double-blind trial, by means of which we can learn what works and what doesn't. No homeopathic medication has ever passed such a test. Where, then, did homeopathy come from—and how could it have survived?

SIDE EFFECTS

Just beginning a career in medicine in 1781, Samuel Hahnemann, an idealistic young German physician, quickly became disillusioned with the medicine of his day. It was widely believed by physicians of the time that a crisis must be reached before a patient can begin to recover—and so doctors learned to be experts at creating a crisis. They treated their patients with purges and bleeding, as well as such toxic medications as antimony and belladonna. It was a very bad time to get sick. The advent of scientific medicine, including insistence on double-blind testing, was still more than a hundred years away.

Only a year out of medical school and newly married, Hahnemann gave up his practice, describing medicine as "the treatment of unknown pathological states with unknown medicines." He even characterized medical practices of the day as "murder." Being proficient in ten languages, Hahnemann began supporting his wife and growing family—eventually he had eleven children—by translating medical treatises.

One treatise described the treatment of malaria with cinchona bark, or quinine. Curious, he experimented with it on himself, and experienced symptoms similar to those of malaria. It was a turning point in his life. On the basis of this single personal anecdote, he declared the Law of Similars: "Like cures like," or *similia, similabus, curantor*. A substance that causes certain symptoms in a healthy person, he concluded, could be used to treat illnesses that have the same symptoms.

The idea was not as new as Hahnemann suggested. Ancient Greek writings contain similar ideas, which he could have encountered in his translations. The Law of Similars is an example of imitative magic. Probably the oldest form of magic, imitative magic is still common in primitive societies around the world. Excited by what he imagined to be a new principle of medicine, he resumed his medical career and began experimenting with all kinds of natural substances, attempting to match up the symptoms they induced in healthy people with the symptoms of various illnesses.

Unfortunately, some of the side effects associated with the use of these substances were serious, bringing Hahnemann perilously close the sort of medicine he had earlier condemned. In an effort to reduce the severity of the side effects, he took the rather obvious step of diluting the medicine. As you would expect, dilution reduced the side effects, but to his astonishment Hahnemann also observed that patients given the dilute medication recovered more quickly from their illness.

At that point, you and I might have concluded that the medicine was preventing them from getting better. Perhaps that's why you and I have never discovered a new principle of medicine.

Hahnemann reached the opposite conclusion. He thought it showed that the more medicine is diluted, the more potent it becomes. He called this the Law of Infinitesimals, and declared it to be his second great discovery. Stated without qualification, the Law of Infinitesimals sounds to modern ears like *reductio ad absurdum*. The obvious question it raises is, where do you stop?

LESS IS MORE

Hahnemann didn't stop; he just kept diluting. He was deliberately seeking to eliminate the material part of the medicine. In his *Organon of the Medical Art,* Hahnemann attributes healing to a spiritual "medicinal energy," which he says is most powerful "when it communicates nothing material." He wrote, for example, that smallpox and measles can be transmitted from one child to another without anything material being passed, comparing it to the force a magnet exerts on a needle it does not touch. This is "vitalism," the belief that life involves some spiritual essence beyond chemistry or physics. It was the prevailing medical superstition of the time.

However, Hahnemann could not have known how many dilutions were needed to ensure that that no material part of the medicine remained. To calculate the dilution limit you need to know Avogadro's number, the number of molecules in one mole of a substance. Amedeo Avogadro, an Italian physicist, was a contemporary of Hahnemann, but not even Avogadro knew Avogadro's number. In 1811, a year after publication of Hahnemann's first edition of *Organon of the Medical Art,* Avogadro showed on the basis of the ideal gas law, that such a number must exist, but it would be another fifty years before Johann Loschmidt, a German physicist, would actually determine the number. In German-speaking countries it is known as Loschmidt's number, which is more appropriate.

So Hahnemann just kept diluting, even specifying how many times a solution must be shaken, or "succussed," between

dilutions. It is now clear that the number of dilutions he specified far exceeded the number needed to eliminate any material
trace of the medicine. But did some spiritual essence remain?

Fortunately for Hahnemann's patients, the Law of Infinitesimals cancelled the Law of Similars. Your baby has diaper rash?
Dr. Hahnemann's prescription, based on the Law of Similars,
would be to treat baby with something that causes a rash. He
prescribed the herb *Rhus toxicodendrum*, more commonly
known as poison ivy. Fortunately for baby, the Law of Infinitesimals calls for a 30C dilution of *rhus toxicodendrum*, more
than enough to ensure that not a single molecule of the toxin
could remain in the medication. If the affected area is kept
clean and dry for a few days, the diaper rash will disappear—
and homeopathy will be credited with another success.

SNAKE OIL

As word spread of Hahnemann's "successes," doctors all over
Europe began experimenting with and adopting his methods.
Hahnemann imagined that he had made a major contribution
to medical lore, and in a way perhaps he did. Although the two
laws that form the basis of homeopathy are clearly nonsense in
the light of what is now known, the Law of Infinitesimals did
allow patients to heal without being poisoned by their doctor.
To the extent that it keeps people from being overmedicated,
homeopathy may still benefit some people today.

Meanwhile, across the Atlantic there was a desperate shortage of trained doctors, even though there were no standards for
practicing medicine. Most doctors in America at the time had
simply served an apprenticeship under another doctor. Itiner-
ant snake-oil salesmen, often barely literate with no medical
credentials, were criss-crossing the landscape of rural America
selling worthless elixirs and tonics to treat every ailment. Their
concoctions were often attributed to Native-American shamans,
hence the term "snake oil" that derives from the petroleum that

bubbled up from the ground in parts of Pennsylvania and was used as a medicine by the Snake tribe.

The belief that primitive or ancient societies possessed magical cures unknown to modern science is, as we will see, behind many other persistent and irrational medical superstitions.

European homeopaths who immigrated to America found fertile ground for harmless medicine that sounded vaguely scientific to the public. Starting in Philadelphia, homeopathic colleges and hospitals sprang up across the continent. By the end of the nineteenth century, homeopathy seemed destined to become the dominant form of medicine practiced in America. But scientific discoveries in Europe and Britain were about to alter the landscape.

Darwin's theory of evolution by natural selection in particular gave rise to naturalism, which a century later would be the world's dominant scientific philosophy. Naturalism left no room for vitalism or other spiritual explanations. The germ theory of disease, emerging from the work of Pasteur and Koch after the death of Darwin, would prove to be the death of such superstitious nonsense as vitalism and such appalling treatments as bleeding and purgatives.

In the medical Wild West of the United States, the Carnegie Foundation chose an educational theorist, Abraham Flexner, to head a survey of medical education. He was an inspired choice who thought: "If the sick are to reap the full benefit of recent progress in medicine, a more uniformly arduous and expensive medical education is demanded."

Over the course of eighteen months Flexner incredibly managed to visit all 155 U.S. medical schools. "In no other country in the world," he concluded, "is there so great a distance and so fatal a difference between the best, the average, and the worst." The impact of his report was enormous. Proprietary medical colleges all over the country were closed, including homeopathic colleges.

There is still a Samuel Hahnemann Hospital in Philadelphia dating back to the 1930s, but the name is now merely a reminder of the power homeopathy once had. Homeopathy has not been practiced at Samuel Hahnemann Hospital in many years. But hundreds of thousands of people around the world still turn to it.

THE TEST THAT NEVER HAPPENED

Some who claim to be healers may truly believe they possess mystical powers to banish illness, but there are many others who deliberately and callously defraud people who are at their most vulnerable. Although the treatments they promote are ineffective, these "healers" often gain a devoted following by simply taking credit for the natural recovery of patients. Legitimate physicians, of course, often do the same. How are we to know whether the treatment should be given credit for the cure? Determining what works and what doesn't is the job of science.

The scientific world was highly skeptical when in 1988 French biochemist Jacques Benveniste claimed in the journal *Nature* that a solution containing a particular antibody continued to evoke a biological response even after homeopathic dilution. If none of the antibody remained in the solution, what was producing the response? This was the oldest question in homeopathy. Homeopaths were inclined to shrug their shoulders and say, "the water remembers." But how does water remember? How can information be stored in homeopathic solutions—or is there any information?

Nature is a prominent, peer-reviewed journal, but peer review does not guarantee that a paper is right. Reviewers often catch obvious flaws in the design of an experiment or in the reasoning used to interpret the results, but the reviewer cannot ensure that the author has faithfully recorded the readings of his instruments. The *Nature* editor, however, took the unusual step of inserting an editorial cautioning readers that Benveniste's results were scientifically implausible and urging qualified researchers to repeat the experiment. In due course some did. Not surprisingly, their results were in total disagreement with those reported by Benveniste.

Nevertheless, five years later Benveniste was back. Supported by the Boiron Corporation, the same company that makes oscillococcinum, he was now claiming to have discovered the electromagnetic signature of an antibody in a solution that had undergone extreme homeopathic dilution. The implication was that the homeopathic "memory" is somehow electromagnetic and Benveniste had found a way to tap into it. He even claimed to be able to record the electromagnetic signature and send it over the Web, making it possible to turn ordinary water into potent homeopathic medicine anywhere in the world. If there was any truth to Benveniste's claim, it was a truly revolutionary medical breakthrough. Such a seemingly impossible finding demanded independent confirmation. Benveniste and Boiron simply ignored the lack of confirmation.

Indeed, Boiron was reportedly contemplating branching out to take advantage of this new "discovery." It was rumored that initial plans called for creation of a new division that would offer instant homeopathic activation anywhere in the world. Once the company had made a major investment in such a plan, I thought it would be unlikely to agree to a realistic test that had the potential to bring the whole thing crashing down. If there was to be a test, agreement on the protocol must be reached quickly.

I drew up a protocol for a simple double-blind test: Ten identical flasks of water, identified only by a number, would be connected to the Internet in any way Benveniste specified. A switch would allow any one of the flasks, but only one, to be connected to the recorded electromagnetic signature sent over the Internet from France. An independent third party would be the only one with access to the switch, and hence the only one who would know which flask had been "activated." The ten flasks would be sent to Benveniste, who would attempt to determine which one of the ten had been activated.

Only after he had made his selection would the independent third party reveal which flask that had been "activated." Benveniste would have one chance in ten of correctly guessing which flask was activated, but that seemed to be the price of keeping it simple.

I tried to reach Benveniste with the test proposal, but was told that he was on his way to Albuquerque, New Mexico, to give an invited talk at the annual meeting of the Society for Scientific Exploration (SSE). I told my secretary to register me for the meeting and get me on the first plane to Albuquerque, and went home to pack a bag. I would meet Jacques Benveniste in person, on neutral ground.

Well, almost neutral. The members of the SSE take pride in thinking outside the box, but more often they seem to be out to lunch. There were talks on such subjects as alien abduction, communicating with the dead, precognitive dreams, cold fusion, prayer healing, and intelligent design. They were all accepted as genuine science—there is little internal disagreement in a community that believes itself to be under siege. Convinced that powerful vested interests, including the scientific establishment, are conspiring to hold back a scientific revolution, speaker after speaker complained that "new science" was being denied funding, rejected by journal editors, and subjected to ridicule—all because it doesn't fit some outdated paradigm. But in most cases it was neither new nor was it science. Most of it was ancient superstition dressed up to look like science. Homeopathy fit right in.

During a break I introduced myself to Jacques Benveniste and we arranged to talk after the meeting recessed for the day. The weather that afternoon was sparkling as it can be only in Albuquerque, so we took a stroll through the campus of the University of New Mexico, where the meeting was being held.

A pleasant, mild-mannered man, Benveniste readily agreed to my proposal to conduct a double-blind test. When it came to working out the details, however, his responses became vague and defensive. He was offended that his results were not simply accepted; it would be a waste of time to repeat the work, he said. After all, why would anyone question his science? I assured him that all this is necessary in today's research environment, particularly when the results hold such promise for the world.

Then there was the question of money, how would all this be paid for? "It shouldn't cost much," I said, "it can all be done by e-mail. You already have the equipment to capture and digitize the electromagnetic signature. Once you have remotely activated one of the flasks in my laboratory using the Web, we will express all ten flasks to you. All you need to do is check them to see which one has the signature. The whole thing should take the two of us a couple of hours at most."

"No, no," he explained, "it's much more difficult than that. The homeopathic signal is only a small part of the total electromagnetic radiation coming from the homeopathic solution, *and we have no way of knowing which part* (emphasis added). We record the entire electromagnetic signal coming from the solution, and use it all to activate ordinary water, even though only a tiny portion is the homeopathic signal. The rest has no effect."

"How then do you know the homeopathic information is in there," I asked in amazement.

"Because the Internet-activated solution is just as effective as the original homeopathic solution," Benveniste replied.

I was speechless. We sat on a bench beside a fountain surrounded by yellow spires of Spanish broom and breathed in their heady fragrance while I tried to absorb what I had just heard: Of course the "activated" flask would be just as effective as the homeopathic solution in his laboratory back in Lyon, but so would the other nine flasks that had not been activated. But Jacques Benveniste had no way of directly detecting the homeopathic signal.

The electromagnetic signal picked up from Benveniste's homeopathic solution was the inevitable thermal noise, generated by the thermal motion of charged particles in any substance.

A brick would have given the same signal. Benveniste had never actually seen a homeopathic signature; he had only seen thermal noise. It was the familiar pattern-recognition delusion we discussed earlier. For Benveniste the signature didn't have to be seen—we would recognize it by its effect. But no one else could see the effect. It was an invention of his brain to conform to his expectation. The mild-mannered man sitting next to me, I now realized, was a lunatic.

What was I to do now? Benveniste was obviously not violent, but he could gravely injure others by misleading them. The media often portrayed him as a brilliant scientist who defied the scientific establishment. At this meeting of science outcasts he was something of a hero. As I saw it, there was little choice but to go on with the double-blind test. It was more important than ever to discredit this madman's claims.

Our discussion ended with us shaking hands on an agreement to work together to arrange the test, but the logistical details were unresolved. Benveniste said he would need a few weeks to get ready. In my heart I doubted it would ever happen.

I appealed to Brian Josephson to use his influence with Benveniste. A Cambridge University Nobel Laureate in Physics (1973), Josephson has a long history of endorsing claims that most scientists would pass off as pseudoscience. Josephson had publicly stated his belief that Benveniste was right, and I thought he would have some influence with Benveniste. Josephson genuinely believed that Benveniste would be vindicated by the test, and did his best to prod him into action. Benveniste always seemed to agree to the test, but would then find a reason why he needed a little more time.

Leon Jaroff, the highly respected former science editor for *Time* magazine, contacted me. He had heard about Benveniste's preposterous claim and my challenge of a double-blind test. Now retired, Jaroff still contributes occasional pungent pieces to *Time*. He made the challenge public in a *Time* article on May 17, 1999. The hope was that it would bring pressure on Benveniste's employers to prod him into action. As always,

Benveniste expressed his desire to cooperate in the test—but asked for a few more weeks to get ready.

Weeks became months. Years passed. Religious fanatics flew airliners into the World Trade Center; an obscure physicist was struck by a falling tree; but Jacques Benveniste still needed more time. In 2004, five years after agreeing to the challenge, Benveniste, sixty-nine, underwent a heart operation. Following the operation, he suffered a fatal heart attack. Jacques Benveniste never had enough time. In this life, none of us do.

THE ALTERNATIVES?

Perhaps Samuel Hahnemann can be forgiven his quaint medical beliefs. When he wrote the original 1810 edition of *Organon*, vitalism was an accepted medical reality. Pasteur and Koch were not yet born, and the germ theory of disease did not exist. Diseases such as cholera were thought to be spread by miasmas, or bad air.

But while Hahnemann can be forgiven, his followers today cannot. They know Avogadro's number—it's memorized in high school chemistry classes. The germ theory of disease is taught in elementary school. Virtually everything we know about the prevention and cure of disease has been learned in the hundred and fifty years since the death of Samuel Hahnemann. And yet, hundreds of thousands of people around the world continue to turn to Hahnemann's homeopathy. We need to understand why.

Homeopathy is just one of hundreds of unproven medical treatments described as "alternative medicine" that are used, at least occasionally, by a third of the population. New alternative therapies seem to pop up every day. Most, like homeopathy, have their roots in ancient superstitions. By omitting the time-consuming and costly step of clinical trials, anyone can proclaim a new alternative therapy. And it can be very profitable. Desperate people will try anything, at any price—what have they got to lose?

The media tends to treat "alternative medicine," from homeopathy and magnets to herbs and acupuncture, as a separate field of medicine. But there is no field of medicine that can be called "alternative"; there is only medicine that works and medicine that doesn't. All that alternative therapies have in common is that they have not been proven to work. There are hundreds of drugs and therapies under development that have also not yet been proven to work, but whose developers would indignantly deny that they're working on "alternative medicine." Alternative medicine is not a separate field of medicine; it's a separate culture—a culture of credulity.

The cultural divide is very deep: On one side is medical science, characterized by an unbroken chain of logical inference based on physical evidence, leading ultimately to clinical trials. On the alternative side, huge gaps in the evidence chain are filled in with wishful thinking, superstitious nonsense, selected anecdotes, and even deliberate fraud. And there are never, never, independent, placebo-controlled, statistically-significant, double-blind trials. Its appeal is to the basic sense of optimism that sees us through difficult times, but that also makes us vulnerable to fools and scoundrels.

BEE POLLEN

The NIH Office of Alternative Medicine (OAM) was tiny by NIH standards, with an annual budget of only $1 million in a $15 billion agency. But to many in the public it made alternative medicine seem respectable. Surely the NIH wouldn't have an Office of Alternative Medicine if there was no alternative medicine? A single line in the report language accompanying the 1992 NIH appropriations bill, inserted by Senator Tom Harkin, a populist Democrat from Iowa, was all it took to create an NIH Office of Alternative Medicine. The report accompanying an appropriations bill describes how Congress would like an agency to spend the appropriated money. It does not have the force of law, but it is almost always followed since Congress can retaliate by cutting the agency's funding in the next year's appropriation. Harkin imagined that he had been cured of allergies by taking capsules of bee pollen, an untested folk remedy, and was determined to make the supposed benefits of alternative medicine available to everyone.

Powerful members of Congress like Harkin, who headed the Appropriations Committee, often go far beyond the report language, dictating every detail of how a program is conducted. The new OAM was initially run right out of Harkin's office in the Hart Senate Office Building. To head the new office, Harkin picked Wayne Jonas, MD, a lieutenant colonel in the U.S. Army. Jonas saw his responsibility more as promoting alternative medicine than investigating it, and staffed the office with other believers.

Described on the cover as "the nation's leading homeopathist," in 1996 Jonas, with Jennifer Jacobs, wrote *Healing with Homeopathy: The Complete Guide*. In an early chapter, Jonas attempts to deal with homeopathy's apparent violation of causality. He ends the chapter by speculating that "perhaps it will all be found to be just the placebo effect." It was only a single line in the most influential book on homeopathy since Hahnemann's *Organon of the Medical Art*, but it would turn out to be prophetic. In 1996 the placebo effect was still largely a mystery, but that was about to change. As we will see in the next chapter, modern studies of the brain are providing a complete understanding of the placebo effect.

The influence of the OAM was out of all proportion to its budget. The movement in the United States toward "natural" or "alternative" medicine was growing rapidly and this was the only office in the federal government with responsibility for furthering alternative medicine. With Harkin's help on the Appropriations Committee, the OAM budget grew exponentially.

As the budget grew, however, so did pressure for federal research funds to investigate the claims of alternative medicine. Harkin began pushing for an elevation of the office to the status of a center. However, the NIH director, Harold Varmus, a Nobel Laureate greatly admired in the science community, was concerned that research into alternative medicine under the OAM did not meet the research standards of the rest of NIH.

To be blunt, Varmus thought it was wacky—and it was. He agreed to elevate the office to the National Center for Complementary and Alternative Medicine (NCCAM), with a much larger budget, but only if he could select a real scientist as director. He got his way and chose Stephen Straus, a highly regarded medical researcher at NIH who had never taken a public position on complementary and alternative medicine (CAM).

In this chapter we use homeopathy as a surrogate for all superstitious medicine. There are far too many CAM therapies to cover in one book, and Straus would have to deal with them one at a time. His task, as with any medicine, would be to distinguish the effect of the treatment from the body's natural healing. But healing is more than the elimination of pathogens and regeneration of damaged tissue. It also calls for relief from the debilitating perception of pain. We will look more closely at the body's pain-relief mechanisms in the next chapter.

CHAPTER TEN

THE DEER

In which the placebo effect is explained

The ambulance crew eased me from the stretcher onto a rented hospital bed. My wife had it set up in the dining room beside two large windows to give me a view into the woods that come up to the back of the house. Since I had last seen the woods, the season had changed from summer to winter. In winter, without the dense screen of foliage, you become much more aware of the animal life. Movements of birds and squirrels on the bare branches of tall oaks and beech could be seen deep into the woods. Beneath the tall trees, clumps of holly and laurel refused to give up their green. I thought the woods had never been so beautiful.

A few days later I saw something larger than squirrels or birds moving behind the laurel. As I watched, a young white-tailed buck with barely forked antlers stepped out only a few yards from my window. I feel fortunate whenever I see these beautiful and graceful animals. Increasingly regarded as pests in semirural suburbs of the northeastern United States, the growing deer population always seemed reassuring to me. In spite of our destruction of their natural habitat by urban sprawl, wild creatures as large as humans still manage to survive and multiply right up to the edges of our major cities. Life does not give up easily on this astonishing planet.

My pleasure at the sight of the deer was short lived; as its hind legs came into view I could see that one leg, withered and limp, dangled uselessly as he walked. From its appearance, the leg must have been injured many months earlier. Otherwise the deer looked sleek and healthy, and seemed to walk rather easily on three legs. Fortunately there are no predators in these woods today capable of bringing down a deer, not even one on three legs.

Evolution has equipped the deer and all vertebrates with natural repair mechanisms to increase the chances of survival in a dangerous world: our blood clots, our bones knit, and our amazing immune system battles infection. Although the deer had suffered a terrible injury, it had succumbed neither to infection nor to starvation, the two greatest threats to any animal injured in the wild. Given time and little else, both deer and humans will recover from most of the things that afflict them, from insect bites and sprains to influenza and food poisoning. Our natural repair mechanisms are constantly curing us of ailments we don't even know we have.

While deer must mend strictly on their own, there are doctors in even the most primitive human societies whose job it is to oversee the healing process. It might not be a Western-trained MD with a stethoscope hung around the neck and a medical degree hanging on the wall, but even a witch doctor with grotesque masks and rattles to frighten away evil spirits can set a broken bone—something no species other than *Homo sapiens* can manage. Archaeologists have found human remains tens of thousands of years old that show clear evidence of bones that had been broken but had knitted back after being set.

What sets *Homo sapiens* apart from all other animals is language. Unfortunately the animal that talks often tells lies. We pass on information about setting bones from generation to generation, but in primitive societies, witch doctors also pass on the rattles and masks that successfully frighten off evil spirits. Science is the only way humankind has found of separating the truth from superstition or fraud, or mere foolishness. In this chapter we will look more deeply into what science has learned about our natural healing mechanisms and the perception of pain, contrasting scientific understanding with the yearning of people to believe superstition.

THE AGE OF BACTERIA

The crippled deer might have broken its leg by stepping into some small animal burrow while running through the forest. It would likely have been a compound fracture, with the broken bone protruding through the skin. A broken bone is a particularly serious matter for wildlife. It cannot be set, or even immobilized, and must heal the best it can in whatever position it ends up. But if the fracture is compound, bacterial infection becomes the greatest threat to life.

We live in a sea of bacteria. They are in the water we drink, the air we breathe, the food we eat, and on the surface of everything we touch. The late Stephen Jay Gould, the famous Harvard paleontologist and evolutionary biologist, once observed that "the age in which we are living in is not really 'the Age of Man,' nor was there ever an 'Age of the Dinosaur.' This is, as it has always been, the Age of Bacteria."

Bacteria took over the world billions of years before humans came along. We treat them with respect, or they kill us. A billion years ago, colonies of bacteria assembled themselves into fortifications for protection against other bacteria. Bacteria on the perimeter of the colony were exposed to a different environment than those in the interior. It was the beginning of multicelled life forms. Those colonies are our distant ancestors. A human being is, in a sense, still a colony of cells organized into a fortification to keep out bacteria.

The perimeter defense for a mammal is the skin, a flexible body armor that is virtually impenetrable to bacteria. However, openings are necessary to allow information to reach the senses as well as take in food and air, and eliminate waste. Eyes are covered by a transparent mucus membrane. It is somewhat less impenetrable than skin, as are the mucus membranes that cover the genital/urinary tracts and the alimentary canal. Because mucus is more easily penetrated than skin, various mucus secretions, including tears and saliva, wash bacteria away and serve as microbicides. Even so, mucus membranes are frequent sites of infection.

Not all bacteria cause disease. There are countless millions of bacteria living peacefully in the gut of every human. They are normally harmless, even assisting in digestion, but if the mucus wall separating the contents of the gut from the body cavity is breached, peritonitis can quickly overwhelm the body.

For the deer, a compound fracture would have provided an expressway for bacteria and other organisms from the forest to enter the body cavity. Bacteria are an essential part of forest ecology, devouring dead plants and animals. Without them the forest would soon be clogged. But bacteria will also use every opportunity to hurry the process along. Any break in the skin offers bacteria an unguarded entrance into the interior of the body.

If the skin is breached, there is a second line of defense. Millions of white blood cells, or leukocytes, manufactured in the bone marrow are constantly circulating in the bloodstream. They collect at the site of any injury to the skin or mucosa, where they surround and devour bacteria or other foreign organisms that invade the body. The white blood cells are aided by components of the blood called opsonins that coat bacteria, marking them for execution. In George Bernard Shaw's play *The Doctor's Dilemma*, Dr. Ridgeon explains that "opsonin is what you butter the disease germs with to make your white blood cells eat them." The danger for the deer was that the sheer number of bacteria might overwhelm its defenses.

I felt a kinship with the deer. My injury had occurred in these same woods and involved a number of compound fractures. My broken femur, or thigh bone, in particular had torn a wide gash several inches long in emerging from the back of the thigh.

It was a particularly dirty injury, with soil, decaying leaves, and other forest detritus in the wound.

In the hospital following surgery, a catheter was inserted through a vein in my arm and threaded over my shoulder and down into the vena cava of my heart, allowing daily infusions of massive doses of powerful antibiotics. Although the antibiotics kept infection somewhat in check, osteomyelitis, or bone infection, was more stubborn. Osteomyelitis is due to bacteria that nestle against the surface of bone where there is less blood circulation, thus avoiding the opsonin and antibiotics. Around metal or synthetic material used to replace damaged joints or hold shattered bones in place so they can heal, there is even less blood circulation. Today, osteomyelitis is a particular concern in artificial knee and hip replacement.

In my case, scrapings from the metal rod that had been inserted through the femur to hold the pieces together were cultured. The culprit was identified as a particularly troublesome soil bacterium. My daily infusions were changed to a newly developed antibiotic that is found to be effective against that specific bacterium. Nevertheless, the daily antibiotic infusions had to be continued for nearly a year until the femur mended enough that the rod could be safely removed. Only then, denied a metal refuge, were the bacteria finally eliminated.

Compare my experience to that of the deer. Although my injury had occurred in these same woods, I was taken to the most modern hospital in the nation's capital, where I was put back together by skilled orthopedic surgeons guided by the latest medical imaging devices. They consulted frequently with various specialists. Psychiatrists monitored my emotional state; hematologists kept track of my blood tests, looking for indications of infection; caring professionals attended to me twenty-four hours a day; trained therapists guided me through rehabilitation. Once home, my wife became expert at the daily infusions and changing the dressing on the thigh wound, which had to be kept open as it healed from the inside out. I had access to powerful pain relievers. Family, friends and coworkers came by to boost my morale. Colleagues filled in for me at the university, teaching my class.

The deer had only himself. The deer's only medication would have been saliva, which is antimicrobial and washes away bacteria. That's why injured mammals instinctively lick their wounds. But how could the deer have avoided the sort of massive infection that threatened my life?

It is likely that the deer's immune system recognized the invading bacteria. Living in the woods, the deer would have experienced small cuts and abrasions that break the skin. Even a small scratch caused by a thorn would allow some bacteria to enter the body. Each break in the skin from which we recover can be thought of as a vaccination against bacteria. The presence of foreign cells stimulates the immune response. Antibodies are produced by specialized white blood cells called B cells. The presence of cells they don't recognize stimulates the B cells to divide into identical clones that produce more antibodies. As the antibodies circulate, they recognize and bind to any bacteria that are identical to the ones that triggered the immune response. Soon there are millions of identical antibodies circulating in the blood and attaching themselves to the alien bacteria. It's the kiss of death. The antibody is a tag, marking the bacterium for execution by specialized killer cells. Antibody production continues until all the invading bacteria are eliminated, and the antibodies may remain in the system for a lifetime.

Broken bones and infections weren't the only hazards we both faced. Neither I nor the deer had bled to death from our injuries. Evolution had equipped us, and all mammals, with mechanisms to stop the bleeding from most breaks in the skin. We will still bleed to death if wounds are too severe, but recover from minor cuts without help.

RIGGED VOTE

If you nick yourself shaving, you probably hold a Kleenex against it for minute to stop the bleeding. Unless you're on aspirin therapy, in which case blood clotting will be noticeably slower and you might need a Band-Aid.

Vertebrates evolved closed, high-pressure blood circulation as an efficient means of rapidly transporting essential substances throughout the body. The downside is bleeding. To prevent bleeding to death after even a minor injury, blood clotting must have evolved at the same time as blood circulation. A balance had to be struck between stopping excessive bleeding and ensuring adequate blood flow to vital organs. Too little clotting and animals would bleed to death. Too much clotting would block blood vessels, leading to organ failure.

But the vote is rigged in favor of youth. As we pass the child-rearing age, evolution stops counting our ballots. For humans in a Paleolithic wilderness, the hazards of daily life must have made bleeding deaths much more common than they are today. Heart attacks, on the other hand, which are primarily a disease of aging, must have been quite rare—people would most likely die of something else first. Today, with life expectancy more than double that of just a hundred years ago, heart attacks have become the major cause of death among Americans over forty-five. We must look to science to find ways to stay healthy in our later years.

JAMES RESTON'S APPENDIX

Many people choose to look back, hoping to find secrets of health in a world before science. What they find instead are ancient superstitions.

On the morning of July 12, 1971, James "Scotty" Reston of the *New York Times*, then perhaps the most important political commentator in the United States, arrived with his wife in Peking, China (now written as Beijing) for an interview with Premier Chou En-lai. In 1971 China was the most mysterious country in the world, having been hidden for years behind the "bamboo curtain." The historic 1973 visit of President Nixon was still two years in the future, but in preparation for the eventual reentry of China into the world, Chou sought to lift a corner of the curtain. His chosen instrument was James Reston, but Chou could not have foretold how it would turn out.

Shortly after his arrival, Reston felt a sudden stab of pain in the lower abdomen and by evening was running a high fever. When Chou learned that Reston was ill, he called on the leading specialists in the city to cooperate in his treatment. The next morning Reston was checked into the Anti-Imperialist Hospital. The story of what followed has been told and retold a thousand times. With each retelling there are subtle changes in emphasis and even of fact, with unfortunate implications for public health in America and around the world. In what follows, therefore, I will rely entirely on the words of James Reston writing from Beijing, as they appeared in the *New York Times* on July 26, 1971, just two weeks after the incident.

Together with his wife, Reston was taken to the wing of the hospital used to treat members of the Western diplomatic corps and their families. At the entrance there was a large sign in English quoting Chairman Mao:

The time will not be far off when all the aggressors and their running dogs of the world will be buried. There is no escape for them.

Even by the time I visited China a decade later, such signs quoting Chairman Mao could still be seen, particularly in rural areas. The Great Proletarian Cultural Revolution had been officially ended by Mao in 1969, but it remained a powerful force until after Mao's death in 1976.

In the hospital, Reston was treated with kindness and professional skill. Tests were done, including an electrocardiogram that showed a slight heart irregularity. As the team of specialists summoned by Premier Chou arrived, he was examined again. The team of doctors retired for consultation and returned to inform him it was acute appendicitis. He should be operated on as soon as possible.

A rupture of the appendix would allow the vast hoard of bacteria that normally live peacefully in the digestive tract to enter the body cavity. Untreated, the rampaging bacteria would kill him. The first step was to remove the source of the problem, the appendix. That evening at 8:30 he was wheeled into a modern operating room, given a standard injection of lidocaine and benzocaine as local anesthesia, and the appendix was removed. He was fully awake and comfortable during the operation. By 11:00 he was back in his room with his wife, where he was given another injection to relieve the pain and a tiny spiral of incense to perfume the room for the night. "Everything was roses," he wrote.

It was not until the second night after the operation that he began to experience considerable pain and distension of his stomach. A doctor of acupuncture at the hospital was called in. With Reston's permission, he inserted needles into Reston's right elbow and below his knees, and then manipulated the needles to get the "chi" (now transcribed as "qi") flowing and to stimulate the intestine. In Reston's words, "That sent ripples of pain racing through my limbs and, at least, had the effect of diverting my attention from the distress in my stomach."

Meanwhile, the doctor of acupuncture held two pieces of a burning herb close to Reston's stomach while twirling the needles. Reston remembered thinking that this was a rather complicated way to get rid of gas in the stomach. In any case, after about an hour he began to feel noticeable improvement, and there was no recurrence. An Alka-Seltzer might have provided faster relief, but we will never know.

That was the extent of Scotty Reston's acupuncture experience in China. He was not operated on for appendicitis with only acupuncture for anesthesia, as media stories reported over and over. He was treated for indigestion with acupuncture, including moxibustion in which heat is applied to acupuncture points—and the acupuncture hurt. Some time later he began to feel better, as people suffering from gas usually do. It was a clinical trial with a cohort of one—a single anecdote with a somewhat ambiguous outcome. That's all it took to set off acupuncture mania, from which the Western world has yet to recover. In his *New York Times* story, written from Beijing two weeks after his appendectomy, Reston clearly recognized the danger of medical exaggeration, but characteristically declined to take a position outside his field:

> *Judging from the cables reaching me here, recent reports and claims of remarkable cures of blindness, paralysis, and mental disorders by acupuncture have apparently led to considerable speculation in America about great new medical breakthroughs in the field of traditional Chinese herbal and needle medicine. I do not know whether this speculation is justified, and I am not qualified to judge.*

THE WAY IT'S ALWAYS BEEN DONE

Always a reporter, Reston was pumping the Chinese doctor for information even in the midst of his own discomfort. The thirty-six-year-old doctor, Reston learned, had not gone to medical college. He had learned his craft as an apprentice to a veteran acupuncturist. Reston asked him what the substance was that he burned to apply heat to the acupuncture points. To Reston it looked like "a piece of a cheap cigar." The doctor told him it was *ai*. *Ai* is most likely *Artemisia verlotiorum*, or Chinese mugwort, which is standard in moxibustion treatments.

I once asked a Western-trained doctor, who now teaches acupuncture at an American university, why only the herb *Artemisia verlotiorum* or its close cousin *Artemisia vulgaris* is used in moxibustion—there must be simpler ways to apply heat? He seemed puzzled by the question. "That's the way it's always been done," he finally replied. It was an answer that applies to the entire culture of acupuncture.

It is also a warning sign. Superstition always resists change. Those who practice black magic take care to perform every incantation exactly as it is dictated by ancient lore lest they inadvertently call down the forces of darkness on themselves. The result is that they have no way of knowing what, if anything, is important. So it is with traditional Chinese medicine, and most other forms of alternative medicine.

It's interesting to compare acupuncture to homeopathy: In homeopathy, Hahnemann's *Organon of the medical Art* even specified exactly how many times the solution was to be shaken between subsequent dilutions (four). Homeopathy today is still practiced straight out of Hahnemann's two-hundred-year-old *Organon*. Since it was written, the assumptions on which homeopathy is based have been totally refuted. Avogadro's number has been measured to five significant figures, and most diseases have been found to be caused by germs. And yet Hahnemann's procedures for preparation of homeopathic medications are still rigorously adhered to by his many thousands of followers. Meanwhile, science has shown homeopathy to be nothing more than a quaint superstition.

Acupuncture is practiced straight out of the 2,000-year-old *Yellow Emperor's Classic of Medicine*, the *Huang Ti Nei Ching Su Wen*, thought to have been composed by an anonymous scholar. At that time, virtually nothing was known of physiology or disease. Dissection of human bodies was absolutely forbidden in ancient China, as it was in Mediterranean civilizations at the time. Nevertheless, the Yellow Emperor's book includes detailed charts showing hundreds of acupuncture points arranged along "meridians," lines that run from the toes to the top of the head. These meridians, which are fundamental to acupuncture, were apparently based on pure speculation. Although every medical student spends hours dissecting cadavers, they find no anatomical features corresponding to the meridians—they simply do not exist. Acupuncture, like homeopathy, appears to be nothing more than a quaint superstition practiced by those who want to believe. But still people report that acupuncture relieves their pain. Let's try to find out why.

POLITICAL MEDICINE

Fudan University in Shanghai, one of China's most distinguished universities, had managed to remain open through the Cultural Revolution. A physics professor at Fudan, who had spent several of those years being "reeducated" by laboring in the fields, explained to me that prior to the Cultural Revolution great progress had been made in modernizing medicine in China, and physicians trained in the West were in great demand. The masses, however, had virtually no access to any kind of medical care. They relied on folk medicine derived from traditional Chinese medicine.

Training doctors in Western medicine would take much too long to satisfy the urgent need. The response of the Mao government was to initiate a massive program of training doctors in traditional Chinese medicine. Not only did traditional Chinese medicine require far less training, it resonated with Mao's theories of self reliance. At the height of the Cultural Revolution, I was told, doctors trained in Western medicine were assigned to scrub floors in some hospitals, while the janitors treated patients. Many Chinese took pride in having their own medicine, particularly after therapies such as acupuncture aroused great public interest in Western nations. Such cultural transformations, unfortunately, are not easily undone.

In 1981, five years after the death of Mao, I was in China as part of a scientific delegation. We had a free weekend and our hosts arranged for us to take a two–day climb up the scenic Yellow Mountains. It was not a technical climb, but for some in our small group the climb would be arduous and was not recommended for anyone with acrophobia. Two in our group did not attempt it. Concerned for our health, the authorities arranged for a medical doctor to accompany us and serve as our guide. Knowledgeable and fluent in English, the personable young doctor was a wonderful companion and quickly bonded with the four of us who made the climb.

The weather had been perfect, but on the second day while descending, a violent thunderstorm blew up very quickly. We sought refuge in a tiny inn that was simply a small cave dug into the side of the mountain with a sheet of oilcloth stretched across the entrance to keep out the storm. There was barely room to squeeze in. Wet and chilled, most of us sat on the dirt floor, but there was wonderful hot tea for everyone. With the storm raging outside, we passed the time by quizzing our doctor-guide about his life in China.

We had not realized that his training was entirely in traditional Chinese medicine. He proceeded to demonstrate by taking each person's pulse. He would close his eyes and concentrate for several minutes as he felt the pulse in the wrist. He would then give a complete evaluation of the person's medical condition, not only diagnosing whatever health problems they suffered, but describing their personal characteristics as well as. Most of it was on target, some of it was not. I am sure he did not find it in our pulses. What he may have lacked in medical education, he made up for by keen observation. In just two days of strenuous hiking our guide had noticed who among us suffered most from shortness of breath, favored an arm, or avoided certain foods. He had not missed a scar or a phobia. It was an impressive job of cold-reading, but I'm thankful that none of us had a need for medical attention on the climb.

When I speak about alternative medicine at universities or laboratories, I have come to expect young Asian scientists to rise to their feet at the end of the talk and respectfully explain that while they enjoyed my lecture and recognize the problem of quackery in Western medicine, they have personally experienced the miraculous benefits of acupuncture, or Chinese herbs, or qi gong. "When we had a cold," one earnest scholar explained, "my mother inserted needles in our ear lobes, and we always got better." "My mother," I replied, "fed us chicken soup—it had the same effect."

ALTERNATIVE POLITICS

Whatever other languages we may learn later, most of us will continue to think in our first language for the rest of our lives. Having few previous beliefs to contradict what we are told, nothing seems implausible to a young child. We really can't help it—our early beliefs are unqualified. We're programmed, and will never be entirely free of the culture we absorb while we're learning our first language.

More troubling than superstitions learned early on is the number of Western doctors that were drawn into acupuncture by fanciful stories of miracle cures coming out of China, and ended up trying it on their patients. Something must have been neglected in their medical education to allow this happen. This is not surprising. There is so much material to be covered in medical school that medicine is taught as if it emerged from a set of postulates, with too little attention paid to the painstaking research, filled with blind alleys and mistaken conjectures, that eventually led to our present understanding. Without that history, students do not learn to be skeptical. We tend to make the same mistake in teaching physics.

Meanwhile, perhaps as a final gift to Senator Harkin, who had been a consistent supporter, President Clinton agreed to the creation of a twenty-member White House Commission on Complementary and Alternative Medicine. The members represented homeopathy, herbal medicine, Reiki, native-American cures, magnet therapy, acupuncture, and so on. In short, the members of the Commission were drawn from virtually every area of medical quackery. Formation of the White House Commission greatly alarmed medical scientists, who were concerned that it would contribute to the spread superstitious medicine.

THE GOLDEN GURU

The commission chairman was Dr. James Gordon of George-town University, a psychiatrist in the fringe area of mind-body medicine who advertised that he could increase women's breast size by hypnotism. Gordon gleefully predicted that the "Gordon Report" would replace the Flexner report that, as we saw in the previous chapter, completely transformed the practice of medicine in America. Fortunately, the Gordon Report would be forgotten in less time than it took to write it.

Gordon had for thirteen years been a follower of the late Indian spiritual teacher Bhagwan Shree Rajneesh, who had come to the United States in 1981 seeking medical care for asthma. His unusual views on sex and drugs attracted a large following, including many professionals whose personal lives had fallen apart and were looking for answers. They purchased a 64,000-acre ranch for him in Wasco County, Oregon, where he established a commune of people who were searching for something. It was legally incorporated as "Rajneeshpuram." Members had to sign all their possessions over to the commune, and spent long hours at hard manual labor as part of their enlightenment. The Bhagwan, meanwhile, was shown on television traveling in a caravan of thirty-five Rolls Royces whenever he left the ranch.

Rajneeshpuram was not, as you can imagine, at all popular with the neighbors in this conservative rural area. After it emerged that his followers had poisoned some seven hundred residents of the nearby town of Antelope with salmonella to keep them from the polls in a local election, Rajneesh was deported back to India. Back in India, he took the name Osho, and formed the Osho Movement. But his health was deteriorating. Ironically, he claimed that he had been poisoned with thallium by the Reagan administration during the twelve days he was held in captivity prior to his deportation. At about this time Gordon wrote *The Golden Guru*, a book in which admiration for Rajneesh alternated with disillusion. In 1990, Bhagwan Shree Rajneesh, or Osho, or Rajneesh Jain, as he was named at birth, died. He was fifty-eight, but looked much older. There are still many followers of the Osho philosophy, whatever it is.

Gordon was not personally implicated in any criminal acts involving Rajneesh or Osho, but it is nonetheless baffling that with his background he would be selected to head a White House commission.

THE UN-FLEXNER REPORT

What the White House Commission on Complementary and Alternative Medicine really wanted from the Gordon Report was respect, but that was the least attainable goal of all. The commission members wanted their pet therapies to be licensed by the state and reimbursed by health-insurance plans; they also wanted to see courses in alternative medicine at prestigious medical schools, and programs to "educate" the public about complementary and alternative medicine (CAM).

In March 2002, the commission issued a huge, rambling report stitching together its various wish lists. The report sought to portray CAM as a well-defined medical discipline prepared to be fully integrated into mainstream health care. Few outside the CAM community were convinced. As Marcia Angell, editor of the *New England Journal of Medicine*, had pointed out four years earlier, "There cannot be two kinds of medicine—conventional and alternative. There is only medicine that has been adequately tested and medicine that has not, medicine that works and medicine that may or may not work." If any of the numerous unrelated techniques that make up the CAM movement had been adequately tested and found to be safe and effective, they would no longer be CAM, they would just be "medicine."

The report advocated spending taxpayer dollars to promote unscientific beliefs that amount to manipulation of supernatural forces to treat serious illness. University researchers and NIH scientists were alarmed by the potential impact of the report, but so far there has been little impact. CAM continues to thrive in our superstitious society, but with limited access to the public treasury.

What the Gordon Report really wanted was for CAM to be treated just like real medicine.

That's what Stephen Straus, the director of the National Center for Complementary and Alternative Medicine, wanted too. But he had a very different idea of what that meant: he wanted CAM to be subjected to the same rigorous testing as scientific medicine. He recognized, as Congress did not, that CAM could not be treated as a field. The only thing the various alternative therapies had in common was that none of them had been proven to work. It was clear that each therapy or medicine would have to be examined individually. It would be slow and expensive.

He knew the work of NCCAM would be scrutinized by the alternative-medicine block in Congress, which had the powerful dietary-supplement industry behind it. The supplement industry had flexed its muscle to get the infamous 1994 Dietary Supplement and Health Education Act passed. This outrageous law allows "natural" substances to be marketed over-the-counter without proof of efficacy or purity as long as the maker doesn't promise to cure anything. FDA involvement begins only after the fact—that is, after the bodies start piling up.

To complicate his problem, Straus inherited a number of CAM studies initiated by Wayne Jonas that would not have passed scientific review. A natural political genius, Straus publicly treated each study as if it was a potential medical breakthrough. That sent alarms through the scientific community, but Straus had to walk a narrow line. To avoid the charge that NCCAM was biased in favor of the medical establishment, Straus sought the advice of CAM leaders as to which therapies showed the most promise. He funded trials of those therapies first, but insisted they be held to rigorous scientific standards.

If CAM therapies were individually rated on "plausibility," they would range from "totally preposterous" for homeopathy at one end to "possible" for herbal therapies at the other. Herbs do, after all, contain bioactive compounds that affect the human body. A few, like quinine and more recently taxol, offer medical benefits for specific conditions. Many, like belladonna, have the power to kill. Some, like oregano, are delightful on pizza. Others, such as marijuana, are banned substances. Prior to World War II, pharmacology was largely based on the empiricism of the herbalist. Indeed, if you're looking for purgatives or laxatives, the herbalists can offer you dozens to choose from.

Echinacea, the purple cone flower, was among the first herbal medications subjected to rigorous testing. A common wildflower found over much of North American, it was used by Native Americans to treat colds and flu, and has a huge following. Although echinacea is not native to Europe, it is now a common wildflower there too, having escaped from farms where it was being grown for the vast European herbal medicine market.

The first results were a surprise even to the scientific medicine community: the popular echinacea showed no benefits beyond a placebo. Over the next months, one favorite herbal remedy after another failed to show any benefit whatever. Herbalists would protest that the roots should have been tested instead of the leaves, or there wasn't enough rain that year, or the herb had been harvested at the wrong season. It was certainly a bad season for herbal medicine. Other alternative therapies, such as magnet therapy and homeopathy fared the same. The lone exception was acupuncture.

IT DOESN'T MATTER

I was the token physicist on the steering committee for NCCAM as it met to advise Straus on research priorities. Composed of scientists from every field, including many sympathetic to CAM, the panel unanimously recommended against further studies of homeopathy on the grounds that neither clinical trials nor common sense offered any promise. The majority of the steering committee, however, thought acupuncture warranted further investigation. I demurred. In the absence of a plausible mechanism, I argued that there was not much for science to investigate. In that, I was wrong. There was much to be learned about acupuncture, but it would turn out to have little to do with meridians or the flow of qi.

It is, as you might suppose, difficult to conduct a double-blind study of acupuncture. People have a pretty good idea of whether or not they are being stuck by needles that sometimes go pretty deep. Although not perfect, double-blind tests of acupuncture have been devised. "Real acupuncture," for example, is compared to "sham acupuncture" in which the needles are inserted in what, according to traditional Chinese medicine, would be the "wrong" places.

Most of the studies focused on the use of acupuncture for relief of pain. Sham acupuncture cannot be used among cultures that commonly employ acupuncture—people in those cultures know from experience where the needles are supposed to be inserted to treat common ailments. But in studies using subjects who are unfamiliar with acupuncture but are told that "acupuncture often works," a modest reduction of pain is usually reported. The reduction in pain is typically on the scale of an aspirin tablet. A small miracle to be sure, but if the effect is real, acupuncture would warrant serious study.

There was, however, one finding from sham studies that troubled even acupuncture supporters: it didn't seem to matter where you stick the needles. What a stunning result. How could acupuncture have been in use for more than two thousand years without anyone noticing that it didn't matter where the needles are stuck? More likely, it was noticed but those who noticed wisely remained silent. For most of history no one ever challenged *The Yellow Emperor's Classic of Medicine*. This shouldn't surprise anyone; over roughly the same period, questioning the literal truth of the Christian Bible could have gotten you burned at the stake. There are large regions of the world even today where public expressions of doubt about the Qur'an could put a person's life in jeopardy.

Since there is no apparent explanation in modern physiology and medicine for acupuncture, *The Yellow Emperor's Classic of Medicine* is held up as the authoritative source. That's a little like your heart doctor citing the Bible to justify his prescription for your high cholesterol. There is an ancient legend known to every Chinese schoolchild in which one of the emperor's guards, who had earlier lost the use of an arm, was shot in the leg by an arrow. As the leg healed, he recovered the use of his arm. This, the story goes, was the discovery of acupuncture. If a more rational explanation for acupuncture ever existed, it is by now buried beneath thousands of years of cultural noise.

PAIN AND PLACEBOS

In Germany in 1897, Felix Hoffmann's father was suffering desperately from arthritis and contemplating suicide. The only thing that seemed to help the pain was the bark of white willow, which had been used for centuries. The active ingredient in willow bark had recently been identified as salicylic acid, but both salicylic acid and ground willow bark and had very unpleasant side effects, and Hoffmann's father did not tolerate either well. Tormented by his father's suffering, Felix, a chemist at Frederick Bayer & Co., began experimenting with small changes to the salicylic acid molecule and quickly hit upon acetylsalicylic acid, or aspirin. It eliminated the major side effects of salicylic acid, but retained the pain-relieving properties.

Aspirin was a wonder drug before the term was invented. It marked the beginning of the modern era of scientific pharmacology. The active ingredient in a medical herb had been identified, purified, chemically altered to improve it, and finally synthesized. That made it possible to produce large quantities of identical material for clinical trials, something that's difficult to do with herbal medicine. Aspirin would be a paradigm for pharmacology for the twentieth century.

The one thing missing to make aspirin a truly modern drug was an understanding of the mechanism by which it relieved pain. It would be another seventy-four years before British pharmacologist John Vane would show that aspirin works by blocking the body's production of prostaglandins, hormones that serve as pain messengers to let the brain know that something needs attention. There are now dozens of pain relievers on the market that interfere with the production of prostaglandins, such as ibuprofen.

There is, however, another and far older medicine to relieve pain. Opium has been cultivated since Paleolithic times. Instead of blocking the production of prostaglandins, opium and its derivatives such as morphine block the prostaglandin receptors in the brain. The opiates are marvelously effective at relieving pain, but have a powerful narcotic effect and are without exception highly addictive.

Assuming the placebo effect really does relieve pain, by which of these mechanisms does it work? Does it interfere with the pain messengers or the receptors in the brain? Or is there a third mechanism? And what about acupuncture—does it really relieve pain, and if so, what is the mechanism?

AN HONEST MAN

For the NCCAM Steering Committee it was not difficult to guess which of the numerous acupuncture studies would find it to be effective in pain reduction. Groups in which researchers had Chinese names invariably found acupuncture to be effective. This "ethnic effect" became an unspoken joke within the committee—unspoken because it can easily be mistaken for a racial slur. It is, however, simply a fact. Randomized, placebo-controlled, double-blind studies may be the gold standard of medical testing, but it was clear that in the acupuncture studies, bias was entering into the results in a major way.

No matter how well a study protocol is designed, there is no guarantee that researchers will faithfully record the results. Are they cheating? Not consciously perhaps. They may be so convinced that they know the truth, that they will adjust the results to avoid "misleading" others.

One of the participants at an NIH conference on acupuncture took the floor to denounce placebo-controlled, double-blind trials as "unsuited to traditional Chinese medicine." The overwhelmingly Chinese-speaking audience burst into spontaneous applause. Their reaction should not be surprising to the reader who has made it this far. Our worldview is shaped by our formative years. Few of us will ever entirely escape the unconscious control exerted by our early childhood indoctrination.

Whether or not acupuncture is good medicine, it is certainly a good placebo. This raises a profound question: Does the placebo effect actually eliminate pain, or does it somehow trick the brain into not noticing the pain? Or is there a meaningful distinction? These are important questions. Fifty years ago it was usually referred to as the "mysterious placebo effect." The mystery is fast disappearing.

One of the groups that could always be counted on for a positive finding when it comes to acupuncture is the Center for Integrative Medicine at the University of Maryland's School of Medicine in Baltimore. Funded by grants from the Laing Foundation and the NCCAM, the center is headed by Dr. Brian Berman, who is not Chinese but whose dream is to find a synthesis of CAM and Western scientific medicine. The synthesis of CAM and scientific medicine is possible, of course, only if CAM works. Dr. Berman, therefore, has an interest in acupuncture trials coming out positive. I do not for a minute think Dr. Berman would let his personal desires influence his professional judgment. However, the Center for Integrative Medicine has a staff of thirty five. As we have noted previously, life is more pleasant in any organization when the boss is happy, and it doesn't take long for the staff to figure out what makes the boss happy.

R. Barker Bausell, an unheralded professor of biostatistics in the School of Nursing at the University of Maryland, was recruited by the Center for Integrative Medicine to apply his skills to evaluating CAM therapies. In his five years as director of research at the center, Bausell came to realize that the placebo effect is far more interesting and counterintuitive than any New Age health fad. He has now written an important and engaging book, *Snake Oil Science: The Truth about Complementary and Alternative Medicine,* which addresses the key question: Is any CAM therapy more effective than a placebo?

Bausell's answer will not make the boss happy.

THE POPPY FIELD

Bausell makes a compelling case that the powerful placebo mechanism is, as he put it, "the body's own poppy field." In 1975, just four years after John Vane discovered the mechanism of aspirin's analgesic effect, endorphins were discovered. They are polypeptides produced by the pituitary gland and the hypothalamus. They are the body's endogenous opioids. An endorphin rush, in which the brain releases endorphins into the bloodstream, can be induced by extreme exercise—the so-called runner's high—or by eating hot chili peppers, which is why both running and jalapenos are addictive. Addiction to your body's own endorphins is sometimes characterized as a positive addiction.

It was soon found that the drug naloxone, an opioid inhibiter used to treat heroin overdose, also blocks endorphins. Moreover, naloxone also seemed to block the placebo effect, strongly suggesting that the placebo effect and the release of endorphins are one and the same. But it was hard to prove. We are dealing with people's perception of pain, which involves all sorts of emotional factors. To be completely convincing, a more objective measure of pain was needed. It wasn't long coming.

A new brain-imaging device called functional magnetic resonance imaging, or fMRI, had just been developed. It allows researchers to view high-resolution, three-dimensional images of the active areas of the brain. To some extent, it can tell what you're thinking about. Used as a lie detector, this technology may invade our last refuge of privacy, but as a research tool fMRI is transforming the field of experimental psychology.

Psychology used to be looked down on by biologists and physicists as soft science. Brain imaging techniques, however, have put the study of human behavior at the very frontier of modern science. The "mysterious placebo effect" was one of the first targets of brain-imaging technologies.

Bausell's conclusion that the placebo effect causes the body's own poppy field to supply pain relief was soon independently reinforced by fMRI studies in which a placebo was found to activate precisely the same places in the brain that are activated by endorphins and other opioids. Depression, even more than pain, is not easily quantified, and studies must depend on the patients' self-assessment. It was found that a sugar pill taken by patients who believed they we're getting an antidepressant not only relieved their depression, it activated exactly the same place in the brain as the prescription antidepressants Zoloft and Paxil.

Acupuncture and other alternative therapies are not, of course, confined just to providing pain relief.

THE FIFTH TOENAIL

According to a report in the *Journal of the American Medical Association* in November of 1998, Americans were visiting alternative medicine providers more frequently than primary care physicians. There is, however, a dearth of scientific evidence for either the safety or efficacy of alternative therapies. This prompted the journal to put out a special issue on alternative medicine research. At a press briefing at the National Press Club in Washington, the editor selected five articles from the issue for review. One of these dealt with moxibustion, which you will recall was used to treat James Reston for indigestion during his 1971 trip to Beijing.

Rather than inserting needles, moxibustion involves applying heat to acupuncture points by burning the herb *Artemisia verlotiorum*. The particular application covered in the press briefing was "correction of breech presentation" in births. In breech births, the baby emerges buttocks first rather than head first. It occurs at term in 3%–4% of births and carries a risk of neurological damage from oxygen deprivation and brain injury. Most fetuses in the breech position get themselves turned around without help before entering society, but often wait to do so until just before birth.

The moxibustion treatment consists of putting a small pile of the dried herb on the acupuncture point, which for correction of breech position is on the outside corner of the fifth toenail. Why the corner of the fifth toenail? Because that's the way it's always been done. The *Artemisia verlotiorum* is then ignited. Just before blistering occurs the burning herb is brushed off. The result, according to the study, was that among women receiving the moxibustion treatment, more of the fetuses turned head first before delivery.

The trial, however, was not blind. Sham moxibustion was not possible since the study was conducted in China where most women know the "correct" acupuncture point for breech presentation. Not only did the subjects know they received the moxibustion treatment, the doctors also knew. It appears that only the fetuses were in the dark.

More recently, a morning news story on CNN in July 2007 promised new hope for women having trouble becoming pregnant. Acupuncture, it was reported, was being used with great success to treat women undergoing in vitro fertilization to increase the likelihood that the embryo will be successfully attached in the womb. Veteran CNN interviewer Paula Zahn asked the acupuncturist how sticking needles in the hands and feet of a woman could increase the probability that the in vitro fertilization procedure would result in pregnancy. "It increases the flow of qi," the acupuncturist replied.

Qi or *chi* is the Chinese equivalent of *élan vital*, or the "vital life force." In *ayurveda*, the traditional medicine of India, it's called *prana*. Acupuncture is said to increase the flow of qi, helping to balance the yin with the yang, which is said to be good though it's not clear why. There is not much point in inquiring further; there is nothing more acupuncturists can say in response to the "how-does-it-work" questions. They don't know how it works. Qi explains nothing. No one has suggested a way to even verify the existence of qi, much less measure its flow. In the language of physics, qi has no metric. The most an acupuncturist can do is to argue that if someone gets better, their qi must be responsible. Don't even ask about yin and yang. Paula Zahn then turned to a "fertility expert" from NYU to see if he could explain how it might work. "We're still looking for the science," he said, "but acupuncture has been around for more than 3,000 years, so it must work."

This unhelpful answer does raise an interesting point. The proper acupuncture treatment for women undergoing in vitro fertilization can't have come from the *Yellow Emperor's Classic of Medicine*—it was written 2,000 years before in vitro fertilization would be developed. Acupuncturists, it seems, will treat anything people are prepared to pay for. They're freelancing, making it up as they encounter new conditions, because there is no underlying theory that would tell them what the acupuncture point should be to get the embryo to attach in the womb.

Astrology has been around much longer than acupuncture; ghosts and demons have been around longer still. They are all relics of a time when *Homo sapiens* faced a world they had no hope of understanding. All the talk of qi and energy-healing and chakras means nothing if these things can't be measured. Neither the meridians nor qi has ever been seen. Worse, we wouldn't know how to recognize qi if we saw it. As we found with prayer in chapter 3, there simply is no metric.

The point of this chapter, and indeed of the entire book, is not that people believe foolish things. Of course they do—it's part of the human condition. Superstitious beliefs often trace back to the first years of our lives, the period in which we are learning our first language.

We saw in chapter 2 that all children can digest lactose. In many parts of the world, however, the enzyme that breaks down lactose is no longer produced after about age four. The child becomes lactose intolerant, unable to digest dairy products. It's a natural development of childhood that allows infants to breast feed without competition from older siblings.

Superstitious belief can also be thought of as a natural condition of childhood. Because learning is so important to survival, the child's brain is very receptive. It is to a large extent a blank slate, particularly receptive to language but also vulnerable to superstitious explanations of the world. But why are some people able to shed their superstitions after puberty so much more easily than others? Does the answer lie in the human genome? Is there a "belief gene" that makes us receptive to preposterous explanations about the world as children? Is it supposed to turn off as we mature, but sometimes doesn't?

CHAPTER ELEVEN

THE MORAL LAW

In which we instinctively know right from wrong

The red granite dome of the Texas capitol still reflected the rays of the setting sun while the rest of Austin was already in the shadows. It was an inspiring view from the high cab of the truck as we crossed over the Colorado River on Congress Avenue. The avenue ran straight through the downtown business district and up to the capitol atop the highest point in Austin. At nineteen, I had never seen a building that big or that grand.

The driver stopped to let me out when the truck route turned off about halfway up the hill, and wished me luck. From the capitol, he told me, I would see the University of Texas just few blocks farther. I had hitchhiked the three hundred miles up from the town of Donna on the Rio Grande River to register for classes that would start in a couple of weeks. I didn't know there was any other way to travel. I walked up through the large grounds and straight into the capitol building to find a men's room. It was a different time. The building was not locked and there were no guards.

Fifty years later, on his way to the law library at the University of Texas from a patch of woods down by the river, Thomas Van Orden would walk up that same avenue and through the capitol grounds every day. Van Orden had fallen on hard times. A Viet Nam veteran, he grew up in Dallas and after the war earned a law degree from Southern Methodist University. Married with a son and daughter, he was practicing criminal law in Houston when something happened. He wouldn't talk about it to reporters, but apparently he suffered some sort of severe emotional trauma, and seemed unable to function. He had accepted payment for legal work, but failed to carry out his responsibilities. A court suspended his license to practice law; his wife divorced him and took the children. Penniless with no means of earning a living, he was reduced to living, on food stamps in a tent he pitched each night on the river bank. He would take it down and hide it in the brush the next morning. On his own he straightened his mind out and spent his days peacefully reading in the law library, becoming an expert on constitutional law.

Each day as Van Orden crossed through the capitol grounds on his way to the university, he passed a red granite monument bearing the Ten Commandments from the King James Version of the Bible. Inscribed in large letters above the commandments was "I AM the LORD thy GOD." Located on the grounds of the Texas capitol, it was a clear violation of the Establishment Clause of the U.S. Constitution:

Congress shall make no law respecting an establishment of religion, or prohibiting the free exercise thereof.

Reflecting the dominant religious concerns of the colonists, many of whom came to these shores looking for freedom from government-imposed religion, this single phrase in the Constitution sets the United States apart from every other country in the world. But it was not until the second half of the twentieth century that the Supreme Court interpreted the establishment and free-exercise clauses of the First Amendment more broadly to prohibit promotion of religion by state governments.

That's what sets both science and the law apart from religion. Science and law are interdependent to an extent that is not generally recognized by the public. When better evidence of nature's laws is uncovered, scientists celebrate the advance of human knowledge and rewrite the textbooks. If existing laws of government are outdated in the light of new scientific knowledge, they are either rewritten or reinterpreted by the courts. Although the law necessarily lags behind the advance of knowledge, both science and the law are evidence-based engines for change. Religious fundamentalism, by contrast, is about resisting change. If new knowledge conflicts with doctrine, it is declared to be false, regardless of the evidence. In a democracy, religion is by its nature inimical to both science and the law.

As he passed the monument on his trek to the law library and read "I AM the LORD thy GOD," Van Orden would mutter, "Somebody ought to fix that." One day, Thomas Van Orden paused in front of the monument and mused, "Why not me?" Van Orden contacted the State Preservation Office that oversees monuments, but was told dismissively that the Ten Commandments monument was not coming down.

REDEMPTION

Using paper and ballpoint pens students had discarded on the campus, Van Orden began drafting a lawsuit to compel Texas Governor Rick Perry to remove the monument. The central issue, he argued, was the government's purpose in erecting the monument in 1961. If the purpose was religious, it was unacceptable. Moreover, the King James Version of the commandments inscribed on the monument omits the part of the Hebrew text referring to God's covenant with the Jews, which made it discriminatory. Brought up as a Southern Baptist, Van Orden had no antipathy toward religion—indeed the Establishment Clause was meant to protect religion.

A district court in Amarillo ruled against him, but borrowing a computer in the law library, he began preparing an appeal to the Fifth Circuit Court of Appeals in New Orleans, which he filed as soon as he could sell some of his food stamps to raise postage and the ten cents per page copying charge for his brief.

Although he lost on appeal as well, Van Orden discovered a conflict between the reasoning in a case the appeals court had cited as a precedent and the reasoning the appeals court used in another case—which it now ignored. The Fifth Circuit Court of Appeals was guilty of cherry picking. In an appeal to the Supreme Court of the United States, Van Orden pointed this out. It was a cleverly framed argument.

The Supreme Court of the United States of America, confirming the principle that all men are created equal, agreed to hear the appeal of this destitute, homeless man. Professor Erwin Chemerinsky, a noted constitutional law scholar at Duke University, agreed to argue the case before the Court. He traveled to Austin to meet Van Orden, and together they walked the park-like grounds of the capitol to see the Ten Commandments monument in the context of other monuments, including those to the heroes of the Alamo and to Texans who lost their lives in the nation's wars. Chemerinsky offered to pay for Van Orden to travel to Washington to be in the audience as *Van Orden v. Perry* was argued, but Van Orden declined, saying he was reluctant to accept money from anyone in the case.

On June 27, 2005, by a vote 5–4 the Supreme Court held that:

A Ten Commandments monument erected on the grounds of the Texas State Capitol did not violate the Establishment Clause, because the monument, when considered in context, conveyed a historic and social meaning rather than an intrusive religious endorsement.

Although Thomas Van Orden lost his suit against the governor of Texas, his teenage daughter, with whom he had long since lost contact, read about the case and tracked him down by e-mail. He was, at least for the time, a happy man. His next project was to find a job, but what had become of him since, I was unable to learn.

On the same day, however, in an almost identical case involving display of the Ten Commandments in two county courthouses in Kentucky, the Court ruled 5–4 that the Ten Commandments would have to come down. The dispute was over framed copies of the Ten Commandments displayed on the walls of two courthouses in Kentucky—and that offended lawyers. Who would want to defend a philandering husband when the jury could see "Thou shalt not commit adultery" on the wall of the courthouse?

The swing vote was Justice Breyer, named to the Court by President Clinton. Breyer apparently based his opinion in *Van Orden v. Perry* on the fact that the monument had stood for forty years without complaint—until it offended a homeless man. Perhaps it had offended others too, but only a homeless man had nothing to lose by publicly opposing this biblical icon in a Bible-Belt state.

The 5–4 splits in the Supreme Court decisions make it almost inevitable that the Ten Commandments issue will be revisited some day. Public attitudes toward religion are changing, and the Court will eventually follow. The change is being driven by advances in science. Let's look at where that's going.

RECIPROCITY

A frequent theme in public discussion of the Ten Commandments controversy has been that without the rules imposed by religion, society would deteriorate into cynical self-centered exploitation. Do people really long to rape and pillage, but refrain only because they fear God is watching? I don't think so.

I asked a friend, a born-again Christian deeply involved in the National Association of Evangelicals, to please explain for me the importance of the Ten Commandments in human society. I think his words accurately reflect the attitude of most conservative Christians: "The Ten Commandments are the standard by which we say which actions are good and which are evil.

I shudder to imagine what the world would be like without moral guidance."

He acknowledged that other religions also offer moral guidance, but he believes none do it as well as Christianity. I should point out that he is the CEO of a successful marketing firm, holds a degree in chemistry, respects science, and is a genuinely good person. I have a difficult time imagining him doing any of the things that he imagines everybody else wants to do, but refrain from doing because they fear God. I don't know what he might have experienced in his life that would give him such a low opinion of his fellow humans.

David O'Conner and Shaun McCarty told me on one of our walks that all humans have an innate sense of right and wrong, put in their hearts by the Holy Spirit. That conforms more closely to my own experience, although I would call that an instinct. I have known some very bad people, but most of them probably knew they were bad. If people instinctively know the difference between right and wrong, then mounting the Ten Commandments on every bare wall in every courthouse in America wouldn't help much. But before we go any further, we should take a look at these commandments as they appear in the King James Version, Exodus 20: 2–17:

I AM THE LORD THY GOD

Thou shalt have no other gods before me.

Thou shalt not make unto thee any graven image, or any likeness of anything that is in heaven above, or that is in the earth beneath, or that is in the water under the earth. Thou shalt not bow down thyself to them, nor serve them: for I the Lord thy God am a jealous God, visiting the iniquity of the fathers upon the children unto the third and fourth generations of them that hate me; and showing mercy unto thousands of them that love me, and keep my commandments.

Thou shalt not take the name of the Lord thy God in vain; for the Lord will not hold him blameless that taketh his name in vain.

Remember the Sabbath day to keep it holy. Six days shalt thou labor, and do all thy work: But the seventh day is the Sabbath of the Lord thy God: in it thou shalt not do any work, thou, nor thy son, nor thy daughter, thy manservant, nor thy maidservant, nor thy cattle, nor any stranger that is within thy gates.

Honour thy father and thy mother: that thy days shall be long upon the land which the Lord thy God giveth thee.

Thou shalt not kill.

Thou shalt not commit adultery.

Thou shalt not steal.

Thou shalt not bear false witness against thy neighbor.

Thou shalt not covet thy neighbor's house, thou shalt not covet thy neighbor's wife, nor his manservant, nor his maidservant, nor his ox, nor his ass, nor anything that is thy neighbor's.

Anyone here ever violate any of these commandments? The first four, of course, have nothing to do with being good—God is just letting everyone know who it is they're dealing with. Consider, for example, this line from the second commandment:

For I the Lord thy God am a jealous God, visiting the iniquity of the fathers upon the children unto the third and fourth generations of them that hate me; and showing mercy unto thousands of them that love me, and keep my commandments.

It's a sort of "love me or I'll kill you" declaration. The God of the Ten Commandments is the angry God of Abraham. But his first four commandments are quite casually ignored today.

God cools off, and in a nice bit of reductionism in Leviticus 19:18 covers all six negative Thou-Shalt-Not commandments with the beautifully positive reciprocal ethic:

Love thy neighbor as thyself.

The reciprocal ethic, or Golden Rule, shows up in the New Testament, Matthew 7:12, as:

Do unto others as you would have them do unto you.

Either way, the Golden Rule is hardly the exclusive property of Judeo-Christian religion. This ethic of reciprocity is a part of every major religion. In Islam, for example, it is sometimes translated as:

That which you want for yourself, seek for mankind.

MORAL INSTINCTS

Could it be then that David and Shaun had it about right? I don't mean the part about the Holy Spirit, but the idea that we instinctively know right from wrong. Holy Spirit notwithstanding, if it's instinctive it must be the result of natural selection, like everything else about us. If we don't yet understand how that could evolve, be patient. *Homo sapiens* have been around for 160,000 years, yet most of what we know about the universe has been learned within the lifetime of people who are still alive. Knowledge begets knowledge, and we are getting ever faster at reading the book of nature.

The source of our ethic of reciprocity, in fact, is just about the hottest research item in the newly-fashionable field of the evolution of human behavior. It involves a radical rethinking of our ideas on morality. The most complete attempt so far to bring together what is known about the mechanisms behind human morality suggests we have had it exactly backward. In his recent book, *Moral Minds: How Nature Designed Our*

Universal Sense of Right and Wrong, Harvard professor Marc Hauser writes, "Our moral instincts are immune to the explicitly articulated commandments handed down by religions and governments."

Governments must impose standards of conduct appropriate to civilization. On the scale of the 160,000-year existence of *Homo sapiens*, civilization is a very recent invention. Our moral instincts, therefore, are those of hunter-gatherers. Sometimes instincts and civilization coincide, sometimes they don't. The courts implicitly take this into account by considering premeditation. We are expected to suppress our primitive instincts, but our endocrine system doesn't leave us much time for reflection. Crimes committed in the heat of passion are treated less severely than if they are premeditated.

Religion, however, makes no exceptions. It seeks to impose laws that are believed to have been laid down by a higher authority. That authority gave us no procedure for reconsidering biblical passages that we are assured were the inspired word of God. Followers are not authorized to revise God's word.

Our instincts are often compassionate. When a bystander dashes into a burning building to save someone else's screaming child, he's not going over the Ten Commandments in his mind, or evaluating legal requirements to render aid, or reciting the Golden Rule. He simply cannot bear to see the child suffer without trying to help, even at the very great risk of suffering himself. He is driven by empathy, feeling what the child trapped by the fire must be feeling. Whatever the risk, it would be too painful not to go to the aid of the child.

In a recent book, *The Happiness Hypothesis*, Jonathan Haidt, an evolutionary psychologist at the University of Virginia, traces the connections of our moral instinct to religion and politics. He parses our intuitive moral system into five moral principles that evolved long before the invention of writing, and hence before civilization. Unlike the Ten Commandments, which consist solely of thou-shalt-nots, the five evolved moral principles are proactive. Not surprisingly, they begin with the reciprocal ethic, or Golden Rule:

1. Empathy—the reciprocal ethic
2. Loyalty to the group
3. Respect for authority
4. Protection of the weak
5. Unifying rituals

All five call for a measure of unselfishness. Unselfishness gave the human race an edge over animals that must survive on their own. We are, after all, social animals, evolved to live in groups that help us through difficult times. Those who abide by these principles, regardless of personal cost, are celebrated as heroes by society. Even in our predominantly Judeo-Christian society, the Ten Commandments are trumped by Haidt's five basic moral instincts, which evolved long before the invention of writing.

By comparison, the Ten Commandments are quite recent, and observed largely in the breech. In war, for example, we simply avoid mentioning the Sixth Commandment: "Thou shalt not kill." Indeed, fundamentalists who trumpet the Ten Commandments most loudly are often the first to call for war. In war, loyalty to the group, our nation, is elevated to first place, and those who are best at killing are honored—as long as they confine their killing to those in the enemy tribe.

There is a dark side. Carried to excess, our moral instincts have the potential to become destructive. Group loyalty can result in constant warfare—warfare between families, between tribes, between nations, and increasingly between religions. Respect for authority can open the door to dictators or that most ridiculous of all human institutions, royalty, which incredibly lingers on even into the twenty-first century. Unifying rituals, practiced at every level from the Mickey Mouse Club to San Francisco's exclusive Bohemian Club can also be the seeds of destructive cults with quasi-religious tenets, such as Scientology.

THE BLACK BOX

Psychology majors have always been regarded with a measure of disdain by physics students. It was a "soft" science, chosen by those who liked science but were unwilling to do the hard mental work of solving partial differential equations. But in recent years, psychologists seem to be morphing into neuroscientists. New scientific tools, adapted from the instruments of physics, are transforming the subjective study of human behavior into objective measurements of the physical entities that define us. Psychology is becoming a "hard" science.

The most basic law of the universe, forming the foundation of science, is that every physical effect is the result of a physical cause—including human behavior. Psychologists had always treated the mind as a sort of black box. They probed it with various stimuli and watched to see what came out. What went on between the billions of neurons in the brain and its links to the sensory organs, to the endocrine system, and to all the other things that make up a person in order to reach an observed outcome seemed much too complicated to deal with.

The analogy in physics would be the laws of thermodynamics. President Bush, for example, announced in his 2004 State of the Union address that the United States would free itself from dependence on Middle East oil by converting to hydrogen fuel, which we will extract from seawater. Physicists knew at once that it was not possible. It was not possible because it would violate the first law of thermodynamics: Energy can be neither created nor destroyed. Of course, all the energy must be accounted for. Some energy is wasted at each step along the way due to friction or some other unavoidable inefficiency. This is the second law of thermodynamics. You don't have to ask how the hydrogen will be extracted from seawater; anyway it's done would take more energy than we would get back by using hydrogen as a fuel. This was obvious because the only product of burning hydrogen is water, which is what we started with.

Why the president of the United States, who could call on any scientist in the nation for help, was not told this obvious truth before his speech is a mystery beyond our power to solve.

Although the black box of thermodynamics was enough to expose the President's plan as a foolish mistake, physicists are never entirely happy unless they can get into the box and see what's going on. The great advances in science come from breaking problems down into their simplest parts, and understanding what's going on with each part. The same is true of understanding human behavior. We need to get inside the brain to see what's actually happening among the billions of neurons, and simplify it to the most basic functions. And that's what the psychologist, having become a neuroscientist, is doing.

THE IMAGE IN THE MIRROR

The problem is that we can't just go poking around in people's brains. But in 1986 a group at the University of Parma in Italy was poking around in the brain of a macaque monkey (that we can do). The monkey was fully awake, but there are no pain sensors in the brain, and the monkey was in no discomfort. The neuroscientists were studying neurons in the inferior frontal cortex specialized for the control of hand actions such as grabbing a branch or picking up an object. They recorded the firing of a specific neuron when the monkey picked up food, but occasionally the neuron fired when the monkey made no movement at all with his hand. They finally realized that the extra firing corresponded to another monkey in the lab picking up food in full view of the monkey being studied. Monkey 1 reacted to the sight of monkey 2 picking up food as if it was picking up the food itself. Because monkey 1's neurons "mirrored" the behavior of monkey 2, they are called mirror neurons.

Mirror neurons are thought to be involved in learning motor skills and language—and perhaps much more. They apparently exist in the equivalent brain areas of humans and monkeys.

However, we can't just go opening up people's skulls, as they did with the macaques. Indeed, many people believe scientists should not be allowed to do such things to monkeys, even if it would potentially save human lives. In the animal rights movement, the tribal-loyalty instinct has expanded to include other primates, or all mammals, or even all living creatures. Ironically, animal rights advocates are motivated by the very thing the neuroscientists were studying, their mirror cells. The animal rights movement can be seen as a case study of misdirected empathy.

Recently, however, scientists have developed noninvasive brain-scanning techniques. In particular, functional magnetic resonance imaging, fMRI, is revolutionizing the study of human behavior. The roots of fMRI go back to the 1938 work of Isidor Rabi, who was the first to measure the nuclear magnetic moment in atoms. The magnetic moment is a fundamental property of the atomic nucleus, and Rabi was awarded the 1944 Nobel Prize in Physics.

The precise magnetic moment of the atomic nucleus was later found to be sensitive to the chemical environment of the atom, which led to nuclear magnetic resonance spectroscopy (NMR). It quickly became a powerful tool in chemistry, and Felix Bloch and Edward Purcell were awarded the 1952 Nobel Prize in Physics for its development. The great advances taking place in electronics and computing made it possible to invent scanning devices that would show where various chemical substances are located in the body. To calm public fear of anything "nuclear," the word was wisely deleted from the name and magnetic resonance imaging (MRI) became one of the most powerful diagnostic techniques in medicine. Paul Laterbur and Sir Peter Mansfield were awarded the 2003 Nobel Prize in Physiology or Medicine for its development. The measurement of a fundamental physical property of matter had resulted in three Nobel prizes and no doubt contributed to the work of many other Nobel Prize winners—and there may be another magnetic resonance prize to come.

When a particular region of the brain is active, blood flow to that region increases. There is no way to directly measure blood flow in the brain, but the paramagnetic properties of blood hemoglobin vary depending on blood flow. Using paramagnetism as a surrogate for blood flow, fMRI scans the brain in two-dimensional slices, mapping the level of blood flow and hence the contours of brain activity. The researcher can watch the changes on a screen as a subject's brain switches from one activity to another.

The resolution of fMRI is not sufficient to resolve individual mirror cells, but their presence can often be inferred. If the subject being tested with fMRI is exposed to the sight of another person experiencing pain, it activates the pain area of the subject's brain—the subject is literally feeling the other person's pain. Just seeing expressions of pain in faces projected on a screen will activate the pain area of the brain.

So now we have come full circle. The psychologists have inferred that the black box of the human mind feels empathy, resulting in our instinct to follow the Golden Rule; and now the neuroscientists have come along and identified the gears and pulleys in the black box that produce this output. Relying on that instinct, what kind of a world is it that we want?

CHAPTER TWELVE

THE LAST BUTTERFLY

In which there is no place else to go

I walked barefoot down the gravel lane through citrus groves sagging with almost-ripe fruit to my grandparents' farm. Both sides of the road were lined with graceful palm trees—except where it passed Mr. Woods's place. Without the palms he could plant another row of grapefruit trees. "How much fruit do them palm trees produce?" he would snort.

As always, the flowering shrubs in my grandparents' yard had attracted clouds of butterflies. My brother and I once counted fifteen species of butterflies fluttering around a single bush. The Lower Rio Grande Valley of Texas was the northernmost range of many tropical species, and a paradise for a fifteen-year-old boy who dreamed of becoming an entomologist. Years earlier my mother taught us to how to make butterfly nets from wire coat hangers bent into a circle and attached to a broom stick with old lace curtains as netting. She showed us how to mount the butterflies and bought us a book to learn their names.

My brother was off at college now, but my grandfather had promised to go with me to find cocoons of *Rothschildia forbesi*, a magnificent silk moth. The Mexican laborers who worked in the citrus orchards called the moth *cuatro ventanas*, four windows, after the large oval spots on each wing that are transparent when viewed perpendicular but are mirrors when viewed at an angle. I still have no idea what purpose the windows serve, but it's a beautiful moth. To get a perfect specimen, however, you must collect the cocoons and wait for the adults to emerge. It then takes several hours outside the cocoon for their wings to fully unfold and dry out before they can take wing.

My grandfather was just finishing the milking, and after turning the cows out to graze among the grapefruit trees, he led the way through the orchard to the main irrigation canal. The valley had once been a part of the vast King Ranch; irrigation had transformed it from thorny chaparral into luxuriant citrus orchards.

The earthen canal was built up several feet above the flat valley floor. Citrus growers had unintentionally constructed a northernmost habitat for *Rothschildia*, a native of Mexico and Central America. The banks of the canal were densely overgrown with willow and Rio Grande ash on which *Rothschildia* caterpillars feed. It was early December, and the bare branches of the trees were sharply outlined against the intense blue sky, making it easy to spot cocoons on the outer branches. My job was to shinny up the trees, break off branches with cocoons, and drop them down to my grandfather. To separate cocoons that still contained pupae from old ones that were empty, we would shake them gently next to our ear. If they were still occupied, you could hear the pupa rattling around.

Back at granddad's workshop in the barn, we built a screen wire cage to hold the cocoons. The adult moths would emerge in a few weeks. I did not imagine that by then my idyllic world would be gone.

COTTON COMES TO THE VALLEY

The Valley experienced occasional winter cold spells severe enough to damage vegetable crops. Rarely, it would freeze hard enough to threaten the citrus fruit and to kill some of the ornamental tropical shrubs, but the Valley had never seen a cold spell like the one that hit that year. Worried farmers wandered among the citrus trees, slicing into the fruit to see if any ice crystals had formed. If so, the fruit had to be sold for juice immediately at a much lower price. The juice canneries were operating twenty-four hours a day, and still it got colder. The fruit began to drop from the trees, completely covering the ground in the orchards. Then the bark on the trunks of the trees began to split and their leaves dropped off. Nothing could be saved—including my dream of studying entomology.

The smell of smoke was everywhere as tractors pulled thousands of forty-year-old trees out by the roots and burned them in huge pyres. Few growers could afford to replant citrus and wait the six years it would take until they bore fruit. They had to plant a money crop to survive. Most chose cotton. With rich river-bottom soil and an irrigation system already in place, high-grade cotton grew head tall and produced huge yields. Some farmers made more money on cotton than they had raising citrus. But the warm winters also produced bumper crops of *Anthonomus grandis*, the boll weevil.

Cotton had been tried in the Valley before, but the warm winters favored the boll weevil and another cotton pest called the pink boll worm. However, the county agent, backed up by an article reprinted from the Reader's Digest, assured farmers that man now had the upper hand over the insect world. A new miracle insecticide, DDT, had just been discovered that was said to be completely harmless to people and farm animals.

Before long, crop-dusting airplanes were out at the crack of dawn before the wind came up, dusting cotton fields with DDT. The white power began to coat everything, and for a time the boll weevils seemed to disappear. Farmers and ranchers began using DDT for everything. Livestock were run through a DDT dip to control screw worms.

There were warning signs. A neighbor put his hunting dog through the dip to rid it of fleas. It killed the fleas, but also the dog. Darwin's theory of evolution by natural selection soon asserted itself. The boll weevil goes though a dozen generations in the course of a single cotton season and quickly evolved a resistance to DDT. It was not unusual to find boll weevils happily drilling into immature cotton bolls with a visible coating of DDT on their backs. DDT was followed by even more toxic poisons. Each would work for a while. The good news, some people said, is that the mosquitoes are gone. So also were the butterflies.

Meanwhile, 1,600 miles away in New Jersey, Paul Ehrlich, a boy a year younger than me, also collected butterflies and moths. But Paul was finding that he could no longer grow caterpillars to get perfect specimens—there was too much DDT being sprayed in New Jersey. It was on the leaves he would gather for the caterpillars to feed on. Paul Ehrlich would go on to study entomology at the University of Kansas under the bee expert C. D. Michener. His PhD thesis was on the population dynamics of butterflies. Ehrlich has been a professor at Stanford University ever since.

The mathematics of human populations and butterflies are the same, and Ehrlich's 1968 book, *The Population Bomb*, coming not long after Rachel Carson's *Silent Spring*, became a best seller.

ENDANGERED SPECIES

By the cold calculus of survival, *Homo sapiens* is doing quite well. There are 1,040 animals and plants in the United States currently listed under the 1973 Endangered Species Act. In spite of wars and obesity, humans are not on the list. We are, in fact, overrunning the entire globe, pushing countless other species into premature extinction by the destruction of their habitat. Even the chimpanzee, our closest living relative is confined to a rapidly shrinking habitat in equatorial Africa and perilously close to the brink. Humans make their own habitat, invariably at the expense of other living species.

The "balance of nature" is a myth. The natural history of Earth is a record of extinctions; that's why we have paleontologists. A successful species in terms of evolution is one that crowds out other species, both plant and animal, by simply multiplying faster. Climate change, natural disasters, epidemics, exhaustion of resources—all tip the scales, creating openings for some species and leaving fossils of others for future paleontologists to ponder.

This isn't some carefully engineered plan. Humans weren't "meant" to dominate the world by some master designer. It's just that, having been handed speech by a roll of the mutation dice, *Homo sapiens* is now in charge and seems intent on paving over the planet, pushing other species over the edge. Catalyzed by *Silent Spring*, the environmental movement resulted in passage of the 1973 Endangered Species Act. Occasionally a highly visible species such as the bald eagle is pulled back from the edge, but in spite of such highly publicized cases as the spotted owl and the snail darter, the habitat of one species after another has yielded to asphalt.

Humans, by contrast, are so successful that we find ourselves spreading to the very edge of the precipice—it is, after all, a finite planet. What do we do now? For Paul Ehrlich it seemed obvious: humans must start practicing birth control. He began alerting the public in a series of books beginning with *The Population Bomb*. We can argue over the details and timing of his predictions, and many critics did, but the end result is inevitable unless we overcome our religious objections to birth control. This is the point at which superstition goes from being a harmless indulgence to a threat to the human race.

RABBIT WARRENS

The technological optimists were horrified at this kind of negative thinking. They believed the world's problems could only be solved with the prosperity brought by unshackled industrialization, supplying an ever-expanding population—it has always worked that way. It's just a matter of figuring out where to put the people.

Thus began Gerard K. O'Neill's futuristic fantasy of the colonization of space. Inspired by the success of the Apollo missions to the Moon, O'Neill, a physics professor at Princeton with a reputation for originality, proposed that the human habitat be expanded into space. He thought we should start at once.

The first public exposure of O'Neill's space-colonization concept was at a physics department colloquium at the University of Maryland, where I had just accepted a professorship. O'Neill imagined gigantic space colonies in the form of rotating cylindrical tubes 40 miles long and 5 miles in diameter, closed at the ends, and located at the stable Lagrange-5 point between Earth and Moon. People would live on the curved inner surface under artificial gravity generated by the rotation. What would these people do all day? Hmmm, perhaps there was an element of sexual fantasy involved. Colonists would busy themselves with making more children, and with building additional space colonies to warehouse the growing population. They would be built using raw materials mined from asteroids. *Homo sapiens* could continue to multiply virtually without limit.

The art of the futurist is to brush off the difficulties with a wave of the hand. O'Neill's talk was focused on the feasibility of the idea, not on the reasons for doing it. For O'Neill, feasibility was enough; like all futurists, he was in love with technology. I don't think Island One, as he called it, violated the laws of physics, but what was its purpose? He confused increased technological complexity with human advancement. On questioning, he acknowledged that he was a committed Roman Catholic and regarded birth control as abhorrent.

NASA treated O'Neill's mad fantasy as if it was a rational vision of the future, funding his "research" and supplying detailed artist renderings of life on O'Neill's islands in space. It always looked like life in the suburbs. The media loved the story. Industry leaders salivated at the prospect of unending market growth. Religious leaders saw an endless supply of souls to be saved. The military imagined garrisons in space, ready to quell any sign of insurrection among the inmates.

Gerard O'Neill claimed that he had run the numbers on his islands-in-space concept and found it to be practical. Worse, he loosed a hoard of like-minded students on the world. These science-fiction nerds are still out there, using words like "destiny" to push ever-more impractical technological fantasies.

O'Neill relied heavily on estimates supplied by NASA for the cost of launching material into space. That was a serious mistake. NASA was seeking the support of Congress to build the Space Shuttle. It employed the time-honored technique of low-balling the cost estimates; by the time Congress realized they had been hoodwinked, it would be too late to kill the Shuttle program without causing serious economic harm in key congressional districts. It was these wildly unrealistic NASA estimates for the cost of launching material into space that O'Neill used to estimate the cost of his space colonies.

To some, O'Neill's islands in space were the gleaming embodiment of a technological paradise, but for others they had the look of a science-fiction nightmare—our beautiful jewel of a planet replaced with giant rabbit warrens.

RUNNING THE NUMBERS

In my class of mostly freshman physics majors, we examine the feasibility of proposed technological solutions to the problems of society, such as the construction of space colonies to relieve population problems, or the use of corn ethanol as a substitute for gasoline. Let's take a brief look at how running the numbers works.

On the first day of class, I ask how many believe that someday in the future humans will be able to travel to another star and its planets. Weaned on Star Trek, most of them—sometimes all of them—raise their hands. So we set aside a few minutes of every class period to plan the trip. Each class period I ask for volunteers to come to the next class with numbers we will need for the next step in planning the mission, such as:

- How far is it to the nearest star?
- How long would they be willing to spend traveling?
- How fast must they travel to make the round trip in that time?
- How many people should be in the crew?
- How big must the spacecraft be?
- What would they need to take along?

Finally, as we approach the end of the semester, we agree on a conservative estimate of the total mass of the spacecraft. I tell them to come to the next class with a number for the annual energy consumption of all humans on Earth to use as a reference point. We are now ready for the final calculation. A few in the class begin to titter, having figured out where we're headed they've already done the calculation. Using simple Newtonian mechanics, we calculate the energy required to accelerate a spacecraft of that size to the velocity needed to make the trip in that period—one-half the mass times the velocity squared—and compare that with annual human energy consumption on the entire planet. The energy needed for a trip to the nearest star in the lifetime of a human—by now they're all tittering—is many thousands of times greater than all the energy that is expended on Earth in a year. So great, in fact, that there is no point in quibbling over the assumptions. It's just out of the question.

The bad news, I tell them, is that we are never going to visit another star. The good news is that they're not going to visit us.

The exercise accomplishes two things. First, the students will never again imagine that a reported UFO sighting might be evidence of a visit by space aliens. Second, they will not take any large-scale program seriously until they have, at least roughly, run the numbers to see if it makes any sense. It's only arithmetic, but it's important that somebody does it. I have never known a reporter to run the numbers; their job is to report somebody else's calculation.

ISLANDS IN SPACE

That brings us back to Gerard O'Neill's proposal to solve the population problem by building space colonies at the stable Lagrange-5 point in the Earth-Moon system. Even using NASA's irresponsible launch estimates, it's impossible to come up with anything approaching the numbers O'Neill used in his 1974 *Physics Today* article on space colonies. Let's run a few numbers ourselves:

- In 1974, the year O'Neill published his *Physics Today* article on space colonies, the Earth's population passed the 4 billion mark.
- As I write this late in 2007, the world population clock reads 6,630,725,709. O'Neill figured 1,000,000 people could live in one his giant cylinders.
- To hold Earth's population to the 1974 level would have required offloading 2.63 billion people onto 2,630 space colonies in the intervening 33 years.

The reality is that the space budget of sixteen participating nations is barely sufficient to maintain a crew of three on the International Space Station. If the ISS serves any purpose at all, it is to convincingly demonstrate to even the most starry-eyed that O'Neill's concept of space colonies is complete lunacy.

Nor is there anyplace else to go. The barren, rock-strewn surface of Mars, like the lifeless surface of the Moon, offers no prospect of self-sustaining colonies. Even if there was another habitable planet in the solar system, extraterrestrial colonies wouldn't solve Earth's population problem. Transporting humans to another location anywhere in the solar system would only exacerbate the depletion of resources here on Earth.

OVERPOPULATION-GLOBAL WARMING

To feed the growing human population, agricultural science created the so-called green revolution. A historic accomplishment of twentieth century science and technology, the green revolution has made it possible to eliminate hunger on Earth—for a time. We need that time to implement basic social reforms to constrain population growth; otherwise it will only put off the inevitable day of reckoning. The green revolution may feed the growing population, but in addition to crowding ourselves and other species out of the nest we call Earth, the growing population inevitably fouls the nest. As we consume dwindling fossil-fuel reserves to generate the energy needed to sustain the ever-growing population, we use the atmosphere as a sewer for the combustion products, mostly carbon dioxide. To feed the population, we use the oceans as a sewer for oxygen-depleting agricultural runoff.

Global warming, therefore, should be recognized as a symptom of overpopulation. We can practice conservation and invent more efficient machines, but if the population keeps growing disaster will eventually overtake us. A growing population simply cannot be sustained indefinitely.

But why must the population grow? "The pill" has given us the technological means to control population. In Europe and other technologically advanced areas of the world, such as Japan, the fertility rate has fallen to two, the replacement rate. Population will continue to grow for a few years because of the large number of women of child-bearing age, but if the fertility rate remains low the population will eventually stabilize—or even begin to shrink.

This has happened quietly without a trace of the repressive government policies that Gerard O'Neill and other libertarians saw as inevitable in creating a stable population. The only government policy on population growth in these countries has been to stay out of the way, creating no barriers to the use of contraceptives. Nor was zero growth accompanied by economic decline as the libertarians predicted. Indeed, the zero-population-growth nations are the most liberated and prosperous on the planet.

Because of the falling fertility rate in Europe, Bjørn Lomborg, who wrote *The Skeptical Environmentalist* in 2001, announced that there is no population problem. More recently, in *The Improving State of the World*, Indur Goklany makes a similar argument based on improving conditions in India and China. Both Lomborg and Goklany are in effect attributing low fertility rate to prosperity.

They have confused cause and effect. Low fertility rates and prosperity simply have the same mother—women's rights. We have only to look at the numbers.

THE NUMBERS

The highest fertility rate of any nation is a frightening 7.0 in desperately poor Afghanistan. But poverty is not the cause of Afghanistan's high fertility rate. The proximate cause is the power of the Taliban, a committed fundamentalist Sunni Muslim movement that controlled Afghanistan until about 2001, when it was displaced, but not eliminated, by the United Nations. Under Islamic law women have no rights—and no access to the pill. The next-highest fertility rates are in oil-rich Kuwait and the other Arab oil states. The per capita gross domestic product in these countries is on a par with Western Europe, but it's the result of a geologic accident. These countries float on an ocean of oil. Once drained, however, the ocean of oil will not replenish itself.

News in December of 2007 that the fertility rate in the United States had grown to the replacement level of 2.0 for the first time in thirty-five years was hailed as an important milestone by the business community, although true replacement would require a rate nearer to 2.1 to make up for childhood mortality.

The fertility rate in the United States had peaked at 3.8 in the 1950s immediately after World War II, but dropped well below 2 a generation later following development of the pill. Industries that had profited during the war saw the drop in fertility as a disaster. One corporate spokesman lamented that "our social systems were predicated on growth—we can't afford not to grow." If that's true, disaster is inevitable. But it's not true.

By giving women control over their reproductive processes, the pill allows them to develop to their full potential. Any nation that fails to utilize the genius of half of its population cannot expect to compete successfully in the modern knowledge-based world. Opposition to the pill is primarily religious, but is abetted by a corporate world that identifies population growth with economic growth.

The pill is not widely used in desperately poor Africa nations, with the result that fertility rates remain very high. Many of these nations are Muslim and suppression of women's rights is imposed by Islamic law. But even among non-Muslim nations of Africa, tribal customs limit the rights of women and fertility rates remain very high.

NATURAL LAWS

Scarring of the skin from smallpox has been found in Egyptian mummies thousands of years old. Smallpox killed 60 million Europeans in the eighteenth century alone, and blinded a third of the survivors. Unlike most epidemics, which disproportionately afflict the crowded poor, smallpox was undiscriminating: five reigning European monarchs were among its victims.

Although a vaccine for smallpox had been known for two hundred years, the disease would occasionally ravage some remote area of the world in the twentieth century. However, an unprecedented worldwide agreement that included every political entity on earth allowed rapid-response teams from the World Health Organization to freely cross every political boundary on the planet without prior approval. It the disease broke out in some isolated region, the team would track down every contact of the victims and conduct mass vaccinations.

In 1979 smallpox was declared to have been eradicated from the earth. It was the greatest achievement of the human race. Not just because it eliminated an ancient source of human suffering from the planet, but because in doing so it had demonstrated what could be accomplished when the entire world cooperates. Hope that the same could be done for polio is fading as religious strife makes such agreements more difficult.

A 500,000-year-old skull fragment of *Homo erectus*, an ancestor of *Homo sapiens*, was recently found in Turkey. The skull bears clear markings of tuberculosis lesions. Tuberculosis was causing suffering and early death of our hominid ancestors long before they evolved into *Homo sapiens*. Tuberculosis can now be controlled with antibiotics and is rare in the Western nations.

But we can do more than eradicate or cure disease. *Homo sapiens* can now aspire to end the historic causes of mass human misery. Hunger is now just a problem of distribution in war-torn parts of the world. Machines free ordinary people from the mind-numbing toil that had been their lot for all of history. All that the world has learned is now at the fingertips of ordinary citizens. What made these things possible?

Fragile specks of self-replicating matter trapped on this strange little planet for a few dozen orbits about an undistinguished star, one among billions of stars in an ordinary galaxy in a universe containing billions of galaxies, chose to spend their allotment of orbits prying open the book of nature. On its pages they found that, for all its complexity, everything in this vast universe is governed by the same natural laws. We can learn these laws and turn them to our advantage, but we can't change them.

As we saw in chapter 2, our search for the laws of nature began 2,600 years ago with the scientific premise of Thales that there is a physical cause behind every event. Science follows the trail back from one cause to another. Physicists are now attempting to follow causality back 14 billion years to the creation of matter from energy, using the Large Hadron Collider at CERN. Much has been learned from the book of nature—but much more remains to be learned.

SUPERSTITION

On the inside we are hunter-gatherers. The brain that enables us to write sonnets and solve differential equations has changed little in 160,000 years. In the scant 2,593 years since the birth of science with Thales, it has likely changed not at all. Science transported us to a world of jet travel and electronic communication with a brain still hard-wired with the instincts of savages who fought to survive in a Pleistocene wilderness.

We are, as we have always been, engaged in almost constant armed conflict, much of it over nothing more than cultural differences, the superstitious beliefs instilled in us as children. Even as science transforms their daily lives, most people refuse to believe that the dreams and emotions that stir within them can be reduced to the laws of physics. A hormone rush, induced by self-hypnosis or a charismatic religious leader, may seem to some to be an encounter with the divine.

Is there a God? As it is impossible to prove there is, so also is it impossible to prove there is not. There is certainly no shortage of people claiming to be in communication with Him or Her. They seem to know exactly what God expects of us, but it's never clear why God would select them, of all people, to be his emissaries. In any case, if we accept the existence of God, we are left with the larger question of where God came from. God, it seems, is not a useful concept.

What science is learning about the laws that govern the universe gives us the power to transform the world into the closest thing to paradise that any of us will ever see. This knowledge did not come from sacred texts, or the revelations of prophets. Science is the only way of knowing—everything else is just superstition.

BIBLIOGRAPHY

Barrow, John D., and Tipler, Frank J. 1986. *The Anthropic Cosmological Principle*. Oxford: Oxford University Press.

Bausell, R. Barker. 2007. *Snake Oil Science: The Truth about Complementary and Alternative Medicine*. New York: Oxford University Press.

Behe, Michael J. 1996. *Darwin's Black Box: The Biochemical Challenge to Evolution*. New York: Free Press.

Benson, Herbert, with Proctor, William. 1984. *Beyond the Relaxation Response: How to Harness the Healing Power of Your Personal Beliefs*. New York: Times Books.

———, with Klipper, Miriam Z. 1992. *The Relaxation Response*. New York: Wings Books.

Byrne, Rhonda. 2006. *The Secret*. New York: Atria Books.

Chopra, Deepak. 1993. *Ageless Body, Timeless Mind: The Quantum Alternative to Growing Old*. New York: Harmony Books.

Collins, Francis S. 2006. *The Language of God: A Scientist Presents Evidence for Belief*. New York: Free Press.

Davies, Paul. 1992. *The Mind of God: The Scientific Basis for a Rational World*. New York: Simon & Schuster.

Dawkins, Richard. 1986. *The Blind Watchmaker*. New York: Norton.

———. 1996. *Climbing Mount Improbable*. New York: Norton.

———. 2006. *The God Delusion*. Boston: Houghton Mifflin.

———. 2nd ed. 1989. *The Selfish Gene*. Oxford: Oxford University Press.

Dennett, Daniel C. 2006. *Breaking the Spell: Religion as a Natural Phenomenon*. New York: Viking.

Ehrman, Bart D. 2005. *Misquoting Jesus: The Story behind Who Changed the Bible and Why*. New York: HarperSanFrancisco.

Forrest, Barbara, and Gross, Paul R. 2004. *Creationism's Trojan Horse: The Wedge of Intelligent Design*. New York: Oxford University Press.

Goklany, Indur M. 2006. *The Improving State of the World: Why We're Living Longer, Healthier, More Comfortable Lives on a Cleaner Planet*. Washington DC: Cato Institute.

Gould, Stephen Jay. 1999. *Rocks of Ages: Science and Religion in the Fullness of Life*. New York: Ballantine Books.

Hahnemann, Samuel. 1996. *Organon of the Medical Art*. Redmond, WA: Birdcage Books.

Haidt, Jonathan. 2006. *The Happiness Hypothesis: Finding Modern Truth in Ancient Wisdom*. New York: Basic Books.

Hamer, Dean. 2004. *The God Gene: How Faith is Hardwired into Our Genes*. New York: Doubleday.

Harris, Sam. 2004. *The End of Faith: Religion, Terror, and the Future of Reason*. New York: W.W. Norton.

———. 2006. *Letter to a Christian Nation*. New York: Knopf.

Hauser, Marc D. 2006. *Moral Minds: How Nature Designed Our Universal Sense of Right and Wrong*. New York: Ecco.

Hitchens, Christopher. 2007. *God Is Not Great: How Religion Poisons Everything*. New York: Twelve.

Johnson, Phillip E. 1991. *Darwin on Trial*. Washington DC: Regnery Gateway.

Jonas, Wayne B., and Jacobs, Jennifer. 1996. *Healing with Homeopathy: The Complete Guide*. New York: Warner Books.

Lomborg, Bjørn. 2001. *The Skeptical Environmentalist: Measuring the Real State of the World*. Cambridge: Cambridge University Press.

McGrew, Timothy, McGrew, Lydia, and Vestrup, Eric. 2001. "Probabilities and the Fine-tuning Argument: A Skeptical View." *Mind* 110(440): 1027–38.

Miller, Kenneth R. 1999. *Finding Darwin's God: A Scientist's Search for Common Ground between God and Evolution*. New York: Cliff Street Books.

Park, Robert L. 2000. *Voodoo Science: The Road from Foolishness to Fraud*. New York: Oxford University Press.

Pinker, Steven. 2002. *The Blank Slate: The Modern Denial of Human Nature*. New York: Viking.

Schermer, Michael. 1997. *Why People Believe Weird Things: Pseudoscience, Superstition, and Other Confusions of Our Time*. New York: W.H. Freeman.

Shubin, Neil. 2008. *Your Inner Fish: A Journey into the 3.5-Billion-Year History of the Human Body*. New York: Pantheon Books.

Silver, Lee M. 2006. *Challenging Nature: The Clash of Science and Spirituality at the New Frontiers of Life*. New York: Ecco.

Sloan, Richard P. 2006. *Blind Faith: The Unholy Alliance of Religion and Medicine*. New York: St. Martin's Press.

Stenger, Victor J. 1995. *The Unconscious Quantum: Metaphysics in Modern Physics and Cosmology*. Amherst, NY: Prometheus Books.

Targ, Russell, and Puthoff, Harold. 1977. *Mind Reach: Scientists Look at Psychic Abilities*. New York: Delacorte.

Taverne, Dick. 2005. *The March of Unreason: Science, Democracy, and the New Fundamentalism*. New York: Oxford University Press.

Trudeau, Kevin. 2004. *Natural Cures "They" Don't Want You to Know About*. Hinsdale, IL: Alliance.

Watson, James D. 1968. *The Double Helix: A Personal Account of the Discovery of the Structure of DNA*. New York: Atheneum.

Weinberg, Steven. 1992. *Dreams of a Final Theory: The Scientist's Search for the Ultimate Laws of Physics*. New York: Pantheon.

Wells, Jonathan. 2000. *Icons of Evolution: Science or Myth?* Washington DC: Regnery Publishing.

INDEX

AAAS. *See* American Association for the Advancement of Science

ABC (American Broadcasting Corporation): *Heaven: Where is it? How do we get there?*, 99–101; *Primetime*, dream healing exposed on, 117–18

act(s) of God: explanations of, the tsunami and, 105–9; science as a vehicle for lessening the suffering from, 114–15; suffering of innocents due to, the story of Job and, 109–12; tsunami of 2004 as, 104–5

acupuncture: double-blind study of, 179; the "ethnic effect" in tests of efficacy of, 181–82; explanations of how it works, 186; modern explanation for, lack of, 180; moxibustion, 169–70, 185; as placebo, 182; as practiced in China, 171–73; reduction of pain from, 179, 181–82 (*see also* placebo effect); Reston's indigestion treated by, 169–70; as superstition, 170–72; for in vitro fertilization, 185–86

Afghanistan, 212

Africa: fertility rates in, 213; migration of *Homo sapiens* out of, 23–25

afterlife, the: belief in, 97 (*see also* heaven); terra-cotta warriors to protect the emperor in, 93, 96–97

Ahmanson, Howard, Jr., 45

alternative medicine, 157–60. *See also* acupuncture; complementary and alternative medicine; homeopathy

American Association for the Advancement of Science (AAAS):
Dialogue between Science and Religion, 8–9, 13–15; scientific community, status in, 12–13

American Civil Liberties Union, 51

Americans United for Separation of Church and State, 51

Angell, Marcia, 176

animal rights movement, 200

anthropic principle, 9–12, 20–21

antidepressant medications, 60

apophenia, 30

Aquinas, Saint Thomas, 108–9

Arkansas Educational Association, 36

aspirin, 180–81

astral projection, 91

astrology, 186

Avogadro, Amedeo, 149

bacteria, 163–66

Bank of Sweden Prize in Economic Sciences in Honor of Alfred Nobel, 30

Barbour, Ian, 7, 9–10

Barrow, John, 10

Bausell, R. Barker, 183

Behe, Michael, 53–54

belief: life of in the brain, 119–21; the New Age movement embrace of, 124; noise among the sensory information that forms, 121–24. *See also* memories; religion; superstition

Benedict XVI, 85, 102–3

Benson, Herbert, 60–61, 69, 77, 128

Benson study, 69–70, 77–78

Benveniste, Jacques, 152–57

Berman, Brian, 182

Bernstein, Maury, 86–87

Beyond the Relaxation Response (Benson), 61

Bible, the: beginning of life and the soul, 86 (*see also* Genesis); the Book of Job, 109–12; divine right of kings spelled out in, 94; heaven, as the authority for the existence of, 98–99, 102; metaphorical *vs.* literal interpretation of, 6–7; the Ten Commandments, 189–95

birth control, 79–80, 206, 211–13

Blank Check, 136

Blanke, Olaf, 91–92

Blind Faith: The Unholy Alliance of Religion and Medicine (Sloan), 62

Blind Watchmaker, The (Dawkins), 38

Bloch, Felix, 200

Bohr, Niels, 129

Boiron Laboratories, 144–45, 153

boll weevils, 204–5

brain, the: as black box, 198–99; mirror neurons in, 199–201

Breyer, Stephen, 192

Buddhism, 108

Bush, George W., 26, 56, 84–85, 198–99

Butler Act (Tennessee), 35–37

Byrd, Randolph, 66–67

Byrne, Rhonda, 124–27

CAM. *See* complementary and alternative medicine

Carnegie Foundation, 151

Carrie (De Palma), 136

Carson, Rachel, 205

Celera, 41

Center for Integrative Medicine, 182–83

Center for Science and Culture, 45–47

Cha, Kwang, 71–72, 76–77

Chapman, Bruce, 44

Chemerinsky, Erwin, 191

cherry picking fallacy, 66–67, 75, 191

Chicago American, 87–88

China: acupuncture practice in, 171–73; isolation embraced by the leaders of, 93–95; Nixon's visit to, 95–96; Reston's appendicitis in, 167–70; the terra-cotta warriors in, 93, 96

Chiron Corporation, 142–43

Chopra, Deepak, 124–25

Chou En-lai, 167–68

CIA (Central Intelligence Agency), psychics and, 68, 91

Clinton, Bill, 174

Collins, Francis, 15–17, 19–22, 42

Colson, Charles, 6

Columbia miracle/prayer study, 70–77

Columbia University, 72, 76

Columbia University Medical Center, 62

complementary and alternative medicine (CAM): Center for Integrative Medicine, 182–83; the Gordon Report, 175–77; National Center for Complementary and Alternative Medicine, 160, 177–79, 181–82; the politics of, 174, 177; White House Commission on Complementary and Alternative Medicine, 174–76. *See also* alternative medicine

conception, the "spark of life" and, 81

consciousness. *See* human consciousness

contraceptives. *See* birth control

"Convergence of Science and Religion, The" (Townes), 3–4

Copeland, Royal, 144

Council on Bioethics, 84

Crawford, Lester, 79–80

creation/creator: the anthropic principle and, 9–12, 20–21; belief in by Americans, 32; early origins of belief in, 28; evolution (*see* evolution); intelligent design (*see* intelligent design); interpretation of the Bible and position regarding, 6; myths regarding, development of, 28. *See also* God

Creationism Act (Louisiana), 37
Creationism's Trojan Horse (Forrest and Gross), 46
creationists: battle against evolution in public schools, 35–37. *See also* intelligent design
Crick, Francis, 40, 43
Cruise, Tom, 117
cultural transmission, memes as unit of, 82

Dalai Lama, 99
Darwin, Charles: celebration of birth of, 55; discrete units of inheritance, speculation regarding, 39–40 (*see also* genetics); finches in the Galapagos islands and, 34; as a fossil collector, 39; Galton and, 64; naturalism emergent from the theory of, 151; religious zealots' dislike for, 50; theory of evolution by natural selection, 22, 26–27, 39; transition to a modern worldview accelerated by, 35
Darwin on Trial (Johnson), 38–39, 44
Darwin's Black Box (Behe), 53
Davies, Paul, 7
Dawkins, Richard, 7, 14, 38, 43, 53, 82
DDT, 204–5
Dean, Cornelia, 20
De Palma, Brian, 136
Dietary Supplement and Health Education Act of 1994, 177
Dirac, Paul, 132
Discovery Institute, 44–45, 47, 51–52, 55
DNA: double-helix structure, discovery of, 40; human genome, mapping of, 40–42; as the soul, 81–82
Dobzhansky, Theodosius, 47–48
Dover, Pennsylvania, 50–52, 107
Dreamhealer, Adam, 116–19

earthquakes, tectonic, 112–14
echinacea, 178
Edwards, Robert, 83
Ehrlich, Paul, 205–6
Einstein, Albert, 129
Elizabeth II (Queen of England), 146
Ellsberg, Daniel, 46
emotions, hormones and, 17–19
Endangered Species Act of 1973, 205–6
endorphins, 183–84
Epperson, Susan, 36
Epperson v. Arkansas, 37
ESP (extrasensory perception), 68, 136–37
ethic of reciprocity, 195
eugenics, 64–65
evolution: Catholic position on, 52–53; challenges to, 25 (*see also* evolution *vs.* creationism; intelligent design); characteristics passed between generations, 39–40 (*see also* genetics); Darwin's theory of by natural selection, 22, 27, 39; evidence for, 20, 42; gaps in the fossil chain, 38–39; as God's plan, suggestion of, 20; Gould-Dawkins dispute over, 14; of *Homo sapiens,* 23–26, 34–35; irreducible-complexity argument against, 53; Lamarckian theory of, 26–27, 48; natural healing mechanisms from, 162–63 (*see also* natural healing mechanisms); Soviet agriculture and, 47–48
evolution *vs.* creationism: in the classroom and the courts, 35–37, 50–55; divine creation, Johnson's argument for, 37–39, 43–45 (*see also* intelligent design)

faith, two meanings of the word, 5–6
FDA. *See* Food and Drug Administration, U.S.

Fermi, Enrico, 7
fertility rates, 212–13
Feynman, Richard, 32, 63
fight-or-flight reflex, 59–60
Finding Darwin's God (Miller),
52–53
fine-tuning argument, 10–12. *See
also* anthropic principle
Fitzgerald, Edward, 107
Flamm, Bruce, 70–72,
74–77
Flamm, Janice, 77
Flexner, Abraham, 151
FluMist, 143
flu vaccine, 142–43
Food, Drug and Cosmetics Act of
1938, 144
Food and Drug Administration,
U.S., 79–80, 144–45
Forrest, Barbara, 46
functional magnetic resonance
imaging, 184, 200–201

Galapagos Archipelago, 34
Galli, Cesare, 85
Galton, Francis, 63–66
Gardiner, Martin, 69
Geller, Uri, 68, 135–36
Genesis: the creation story, 28 (*See
also* creation/creator); the soul,
beginning of, 86
genetics: mapping of the human
genome, 40–42; Mendel's work
establishing the field of, 39–40;
structure of DNA, discovery of,
40; synthetic chromosome to
produce a life form, 103
Gere, Richard, 99
Ghazali, Abu Hamid al-, 107
Global Consciousness Project,
139–40
global warming, 211
God: acts of (*see* act(s) of God); in
the classroom, 29; as collective
term for imperfectly understood

nature, 11; conception as compelling belief in, 81; eclipses and
beliefs regarding, 31; inability to
know the reasons of, 11; as not a
useful concept, 215; testing of Job
by, 109–12
"God of the gaps," 39
Goklany, Indur, 212
Gordon, James, 175–76
Gould, Stephen Jay, 13–14, 163
Graham, Billy, 6
green revolution, 211
Gross, Paul, 46

Hager, David, 80
Haggard, Ted, 100
Hahnemann, Samuel, 147–50, 157,
171
Haidt, Jonathan, 196–97
Harkin, Tom, 158–59, 174
Hauser, Marc, 196
health: acupuncture (*see* acupuncture);
alternative medicine, 157–60;
clinical trials of new medicines,
57–58; complementary and
alternative medicine (*see*
complementary and alternative
medicine); dream healing, fraudulent, 116–19; homeopathy (*see*
homeopathy); medical statistics,
origin of the field of, 63–64;
natural healing mechanisms (*see*
natural healing mechanisms);
prayer and (*see* prayer); primitive/
ancient medical cures, belief in,
150–51; the relaxation response
as antidote to stress, 60–62;
religion prescribed for medical
problems, 61–62
Healy, Bernadine, 41
heaven: Benedict XVI on eternal life,
102–3; the Bible as basis for
belief in, 97–99, 102; mass
suicide as route to, 97; near-death
experiences of, 101–2; public

belief in, 100; sovereign authority in China mandated by, 95; television program on, 99–101. *See also* afterlife, the

Heaven: Where is it? How do we get there? (ABC), 99–101

Heaven's Gate, 97

Heisenberg, Werner, 129, 131–32

Hinduism, 107–8

Hitler, Adolf, 132

Hoffmann, Felix, 180

homeopathy: as alternative medicine, 157; in America, 151–52; dilution of medications, 145–46, 148–50; further studies of dropped, 179; medications exempted from FDA oversight, 144–45; origin of, 147–50; oscillococcinum as alternative to flu vaccine, 143–47; as placebo effect, 146–47, 159; proposed test of claims for, 152–57; as superstition, 171; as "totally preposterous," 178

Homo sapiens: creation myths as superstition among, 28; early evolution of, 23–26; the fight-or-flight reflex in, 59–60; language as the distinguishing characteristic of, 162; limited evolutionary change of, 34–35, 215; science and the aspirations of, 214–15; success of and population growth, 205–6 (*see also* population, growth of human)

hormones: antidepressants and, 60; cortisol and the fight-or-flight reflex, 59–60; emotions and, 17–19

Horvath, Joseph, 76

human consciousness: ESP, experiments in, 136–37; Global Consciousness Project, 139–40; PEAR lab's experiments into the effects of, 137–40; Schmidt's

experiments into the effects of, 135–36; universal, 134–35

human sexuality and development: birth control and population growth, 206, 211–13; conception and the "divine spark" of life, 81; embryonic stem cells in, 83–85; memories from the womb and past lives, 86–89; Plan B contraceptive controversy, 79–80; *in vitro* fertilization (IVF), 83, 185–86

Huxley, Thomas, 27

hypothalamus, the, 59

Icons of Evolution: Science or Myth (Wells), 47

imitative magic, 148

influenza, 142–43

Inherit the Wind, 36

Institute for Genome Research, The, 41

intelligent design: the anthropic principle as evidence for, 10–12; Bush as proponent of, 26, 28; deception to promote, 44–45, 47–49, 55; evolution as challenge to, emergence of, 27 (*see also* evolution); inconvenient truths behind the campaign to promote, 45–47; the *Kitzmiller* case and, 51–55; origins of the argument for, 37–39, 43–44; Polkinghorne-Weinberg debate regarding, 9–10; religious zealots as danger to strategy of, 50–52; as strategy in war against evolution, 28–29, 44–45

in vitro fertilization (IVF), 83, 185–86

irreducible-complexity argument, 53

Islamic societies: anti-American conspiracy theories in, 105–6; explaining acts of God in, 105–7; fertility rates and women's treatment in, 212–13

J. Craig Venter Institute, 103
Jacobs, Jennifer, 159
Jahn, Robert G., 129–30, 134, 137, 140–41
Jaroff, Leon, 156
Job, God's testing of, 109–12
Johnson, Phillip, 37–38, 43–45, 51
Johnson, Samuel, 118
John Templeton Foundation, 2, 8, 14–15, 69
Jonas, Wayne, 159, 177
Jones, John E., III, 52, 54–55, 99
Josephson, Brian, 156
Journal of Reproductive Medicine, 70, 72–73, 75–77

Kitzmiller, Tammy, 51
Kitzmiller v. Dover Area School District, 51–55, 99

lactose tolerance, 24–26
Lamarck, Jean-Baptiste, 26–27, 48
Laterbur, Paul, 200
laws of nature. *See* naturalism
Lederman, Leon, 21
Lewis, C. S., 16–17, 44
life: creation of artificial form of, 103. *See also* soul, the
Lobo, Rugerio, 71, 76
Lomborg, Bjørn, 212
Loschmidt, Johann, 149
Lysenko, Trofim, 47–48

MacDougall, Duncan, 90
MacLellan Foundation, 45
Maimonides, Moses, 108–9
Mansfield, Sir Peter, 200
Mao Zedong, 93–96, 168, 172
Marburger, John, 26, 84
materialism, 44
McCarrick, Cardinal Theodore, 100
McCarty, Shaun: Barbara Walters special on heaven, discussion of, 100–101; contraception, the soul and, 80–82; evolution, the

Catholic Church's position on, 52–53; on God's ways, 11, 74–75; innate sense of right and wrong all humans have, 193, 195; as witness to author's injury, vii–viii
McClellan, Scott, 46
McGrew, Lydia, 11
McGrew, Timothy, 10–11
measurement, dilemma of and Heisenberg's uncertainty principle, 131–32
meditation, 61
memes, 82
memories: filling gaps in sensory information with, 121–22; of near-death experiences, 101–2; past-life regression, 86–88; retention in the brain, 120; womb, 89
Mencken, H. L., 15
Mendel, Gregor, 39–40
Meyer, Stephen, 44–45
Michener, C. D., 205
Miller, Ken, 52–54
Mind-Body Medical Institute, 69
MIT Alumni Journal, 4
Mitchell, Edgar, 136–37
mitosis, 82
Moon, Reverend Sun Myung, 48
moral law: concept of, 17; empathy in the human mind, 201; as innate moral instincts, 195–97; as reason for Collins' religious conversion, 21–22, the Ten Commandments, 189–95
Mother Theresa, 6
moxibustion, 169–70, 185
Muncaster, Ralph, 98
Murphy, Bridey, 86–88
mysticism, New Age. *See* New Age movement

NASA (National Aeronautics and Space Agency), 207–8
Nash, John, 30

National Association of Evangelicals, 100, 192

National Center for Complementary and Alternative Medicine (NCCAM), 160, 177–79, 181–82

National Center for Science Education, 51

National Day of Prayer and Remembrance, 56, 62

National Medal of Science, 3

natural disasters. *See* act(s) of God

natural healing mechanisms: bacteria, defense against, 163–66; blood clotting, 166–67; invertebrates equipped with, 162

naturalism: as basic assumption of science, 5, 44; Darwin's contribution to, 151; evolution by natural selection as beginning of, 27; human advantage through, potential for, 213–15; patience advised by, 21; Weinberg's, 9

natural law, Judeo-Christian theology and, 108–9

NCCAM. *See* National Center for Complementary and Alternative Medicine

near-death experiences, 101–2. *See also* out-of-body experiences

New Age movement: appeal of, 119; belief in, role of, 124; books, 124–25; dream healing and, 116–19; quantum mechanics and, 128, 133–34; *The Secret* as positive thought and tired clichés, 125–28

9/11 terrorist attacks, 56

Nixon, Richard, 95–96

Nobel, Alfred, 30

Nobel Prize, 2–3, 9, 132, 200

Nymphalis antiopa, 1

OAM. *See* Office of Alternative Medicine

O'Connor, David: Barbara Walters special on heaven, discussion of, 100–101; conception, the soul and, 80–82; evolution, the Catholic Church's position on, 52–53; on God's ways, 11, 74; innate sense of right and wrong all humans have, 193, 195; as witness to author's injury, vii–viii

Office of Alternative Medicine (OAM), 158–60

Of Pandas and People, 50

Ohio Board of Education, 55

O'Neill, Gerard K., 207–8, 210–11

Organon of the Medical Art (Hahnemann), 149, 157, 159, 171

oscillococcinum, 143–47

Osho Movement, 175–76

osteomyelitis, 165

out-of-body experiences, 90–92. *See also* near-death experiences

oxytocin, 19

pain, relief of, 179–82. *See also* placebo effect

Paley, William, 38

past-life regression, 86–88

patterns, human ability to make sense of, 29–30

Peale, Norman Vincent, 127–28

PEAR. *See* Princeton Engineering Anomalies Research lab

peer review, 73

Perry, Rick, 190–91

pheromones, 18–19

placebo effect: clinical trials of new medicines and, 57–58; doctor exploitation of in treating patients, 58; endorphins as the mechanism for, 183–84; of herbal remedies, 178; homeopathic medicine, 146–47, 159; pain reduction by, 181–84

Polkinghorne, Sir John, 9–10

population, growth of human: birth control needed in response to, 206, 211–13; impossibility of sustaining, 211; space colonies in response to, 206–8, 210; women's rights and, 212–13
Population Bomb, The (Ehrlich), 205–6
Powell, Michael, 38, 43
Power of Positive Thinking, The (Peale), 127
prayer: deception in the "Columbia miracle study," 70–77; definition of, 58, 78; as a form of meditation, 61; intercessory, studies of efficacy of, 62–63, 65–67, 69–70, 77–78; measuring, impossibility of, 78; as medical therapy, 57–58, 62–63; 9/11 terrorist attacks and, 56; pain, seeking relief from, 62
Princeton Engineering Anomalies Research (PEAR) lab, 129, 137–40
Princeton University, 129–30
psychokinesis, 135–40
public opinion: biblical account of creation, belief in, 49; compartmentalization of, 49–50; dinosaurs, age of, 49–50; God, belief in, 32; heaven and the afterlife, belief in, 97, 100; polls, limits of, 49–50
Purcell, Edward, 200
Puthoff, Harold, 68, 136

Qin Shi Huang, 93, 96–97
quantum physics: Heisenberg's uncertainty principle, 131–32; the New Age movement and, 128, 133–34; at Princeton University, 130; Schrödinger's wave equation, 130–33; universal consciousness/ psychokinesis and, 134–40

Rabi, Isidor, 200
Radford, Tim, 3

Rajneesh, Bhagwan Shree, 175–76
Randi, James, 68
random number generators (RNGs), 135–40
Reagan, Ronald, 3, 127
recovered-memory therapy, 89
reincarnation, 108
relaxation response, the, 60–62, 128
Relaxation Response, The (Benson), 60–61
religion: beliefs regarding, compartmentalization of, 49–50; birth control, opposition to, 206, 212–13; change, resistance to, 190; evolution supported by rational churchgoers, 55; "faith" as used in, 6; fanatics, actions of, 8; as a medical cure, 61–62 (*see also* prayer); science and (*see* science and religion); scientific explanations of, 19–20
remote viewing, 68
Reston, James, 167–70
RNG. *See* random number generators
Robertson, Pat, 106–7
Roman Catholic Church: eternal life, Benedict XVI on, 102–3; evolution, position on, 52–53; heaven, belief regarding, 100; science in modern times, receptivity to, 81; the soul, conception and, 86
Rothschildia forbesi, 202–3
Ruloff, Walt, 20
Russia, Lysenko's control of agriculture in, 47–48

sacred dishonesty: Ruloff's, 19–20; in the war against Darwinism, 29, 48–49
Safire, William, 109
Sagan, Carl, 73
Samuel Hahnemann Hospital, 151–52
Schmidt, Helmut, 135–36

Schrödinger, Erwin Rudolf Josef Alexander, 130–33
science: the birth and essential features of, 30–33; the Bush administration and, 84; consciousness as superstition of, 141; evolution's status in, 26–27, 42 (*see also* evolution); human aspirations, science and the pursuit of, 214–15; intelligent design's status in, 26, 44; the New Age movement and, 128; quantum physics (*see* quantum physics); superstition, as the opposite of/antidote for, 32, 162–63 (*see also* superstition). *See also* scientists
Science, 12–13
science and religion: antipathy between, 3–5; authority, tension between and the appeal to, 99; change, relationship to as basis of distinction between, 189–90; dialog between, Templeton's purchase of, 7–9; "faith" used differently in, 5–6; "separate but equal" as Gould's view of, 13; Townes as exception to tension between, 3–5. *See also* evolution *vs.* creationism
Science & Spirit, 8
scientific materialism, 44
scientists: metaphorical interpretation of the Bible by, 6–7; natural disasters as experiments for, 112; religious, 4, 6, 15, 19–20; religious conversion of, reasons for, 20–22. *See also* science
Scientology, 197
Scopes, John, 35–36
Scopes "monkey trial," 35–36
Search for Bridey Murphy, The (Bernstein), 87
Secret, The (Byrne), 124–28
Selfish Gene, The (Dawkins), 43, 82
sexuality. *See* human sexuality and development

Shaw, George Bernard, 164
Shriver, Maria, 99
Silent Spring (Carson), 205–6
Sloan, Richard, 62
smallpox, 213–14
Smythe, William, 3
Society for Scientific Exploration (SSE), 154
sonar operators, testing of, 122
soul, the, 81–82, 85–86, 90–92. *See also* heaven
sovereign authority, of kings and emperors, 94–95
space colonization, 207–10
Spielberg, Steven, 117
Stanford Research Institute, 68
Stem Cell Research Enhancement Act of 2006, 85
stem cells, 82–85
Steptoe, Patrick, 83
Straus, Stephen, 160, 177
suffering of innocents. *See* act(s) of God
superstition: belief in prayer for healing as, 62; childhood, as a natural condition of, 187; compartmentalization as essential to beliefs in, 50; "consciousness" as science's, 141; creation myths, 28; eclipse myths, 30–31; medical, 151, 170–72 (*see also* acupuncture; complementary and alternative medicine; homeopathy); New Age, 119 (*see also* New Age movement); persistence of belief in, 33; personal, origin of, 121; religious, belief in, 118; science as the opposite of/antidote for, 32, 162–63, 215; threat to human race, religious objection to birth control as, 206 (*see also* population, growth of human)
Supreme Court, United States, 191–92

Targ, Elizabeth, 67, 69
Targ, Russell, 68–69, 136

Targ, William, 69
telekinesis, 135–40
Templeton, Sir John, 2–3, 7–9,
    12–15, 69
Templeton Foundation. *See* John
    Templeton Foundation
Templeton Prize for Progress Toward
    Research or Discoveries about
    Spiritual Realities, 2, 4–7, 9–10
Ten Commandments, the, 189–95
Texas, University of, 189–92
Texas-sharpshooter fallacy, 11,
    67–68, 75
Thales of Mellitus, 31–32, 214–15
Think, 4
Thomas Moore Law Center, 51
Thompson, Tommy, 143
Tighe, Virginia, 86–88
Tillich, Paul, 49
Tipler, Frank, 10
Tishkoff, Sarah, 23–25
Townes, Charles, 1–6, 13
Townes, Henry, 2
Trudeau, Gary, 125
Trujillo, Cardinal Alfonso López, 85
tsunami of 2004, 104–9, 112–15

Unification Church, 48
universal consciousness, 134–35. *See
    also* psychokinesis

Vane, John, 181, 183
Van Orden, Thomas, 188–91
Van Orden v. Perry, 191–92
Varmus, Harold, 84, 160
Venter, J. Craig, 41–42, 103
Venter Institute. *See* J. Craig Venter
    Institute
Vestrup, Eric, 11
vitalism, 81, 149, 151, 157

Walters, Barbara, 99–101
Watson, James, 15, 40–43
Wedge, The, 46, 50
Weinberg, Steven, 5, 9–10
Wells, Jonathon, 47–48
White, Tim, 24
White House Commission on
    Complementary and Alternative
    Medicine, 174–76
Winfrey, Oprah, 126
Wirth, Daniel P., 71–72, 75–77
women's rights, 212–13
Wood, Susan, 79–80
World Health Organization, 213–14

*Yellow Emperor's Classic of Medicine,
    The,* 171, 179–80, 186

Zhan, Paula, 186
zygotes, 81–82, 85